1/19

THE PRESENT HEART

ALSO BY POLLY YOUNG-EISENDRATH, PhD

The Self-Esteem Trap: Raising Confident and Compassionate Kids in an Age of Self-Importance

Women and Desire: Beyond Wanting to Be Wanted

The Resilient Spirit: Transforming Suffering into Insight and Renewal

You're Not What I Expected: Love After the Romance Has Ended

The Cambridge Companion to Jung (coeditor)

Awakening and Insight: Zen Buddhism and Psychotherapy (coeditor)

The Psychology of Mature Spirituality: Integrity, Wisdom, Transcendence (coeditor)

Gender and Desire: Uncursing Pandora

Awakening to Zen: The Teachings of Roshi Philip Kapleau (coeditor)

Jung's Self Psychology: A Constructivist Perspective (coauthor)

Female Authority: Empowering Women through Psychotherapy (coauthor)

The Book of the Self: Person, Pretext, and Process (coeditor)

Hags and Heroes: A Feminist Approach to Jungian Psychotherapy with Couples

THE
PRESENT
HEART

A Memoir of Love, Loss, and Discovery

Polly Young-Eisendrath, PhD

RODALE.

Internet addresses and telephone numbers given in this book were accurate at the time it went to press.

© 2014 by Polly Young-Eisendrath

Rodale books may be purchased for business or promotional use or for special sales. For information, please write to: Special Markets Department, Rodale Inc., 733 Third Avenue, New York, NY 10017

Printed in the United States of America
Rodale Inc. makes every effort to use acid-free ♾, recycled paper ♻.

Excerpt from "Oddjob, A Bull Terrier" from *Selected Poems* by Derek Walcott, edited by Edward Baugh. Copyright © 2007 by Derek Walcott. Reprinted by permission of Farrar, Straus and Giroux, LLC.

Excerpt from *Zen Flesh, Zen Bones* reprinted by permission of Tuttle Publishing.

Book design by Kara Plikaitis

Library of Congress Cataloging-in-Publication Data is on file with the publisher.
ISBN 978–1–60961–360–0

Distributed to the trade by Macmillan
2   4   6   8   10   9   7   5   3   1   hardcover

We inspire and enable people to improve their lives and the world around them.
rodalebooks.com

For Edward Epstein
LOVE ALWAYS

... and whether we bear it for beast,

for child, for woman, or friend,

it is the one love, it is the same,

and it is blest

deepest by loss

it is blest, it is blest.

———————————————

—from "Oddjob, a Bull Terrier" by Derek Walcott

Prologue

In December 2009 I am flying to London from Johannesburg, South Africa, running a high fever. I am in a state of otherworldliness, confused and sick. I've been away for 3 weeks, and the alluringly foreign sights and smells and settings of Johannesburg, Cape Town, Free State, and the Drakensberg Mountains have made me unfamiliar to myself. My return flight has also been delayed by 12 hours and my body is hot and achy while my mind races.

Several years before, I lost my husband, the love of my life, to a tragic illness. Now I am returning home after spending a lively visit with a man with whom I have been having a long-distance relationship. I wonder if I am in love again. Perhaps I have found the thread I am looking for. I'm not sure. It was crazy to come all the way to South Africa seeking an intimate relationship. Something ineluctable is driving me. I've come to find again the kind of love that allowed me to relax and know myself in exactly the same fresh and tactile way I know the natural world around me: the blade of grass, the sun's heat, the smell of soil. Ed Epstein was my best friend and partner. Inside our love I learned how to be curious and compassionate with the puzzle that I am. We had developed the capacity to know each other just as we were and to accept each other without trying to change anything. We never lost the desire to be physically and emotionally close even though we bickered a lot. And we didn't just live together in family and home; we often worked together as couples therapists. Before knowing Ed, I did not know that such a love was possible, and now, after living with him for decades, I do not want to live without it. I wrestle with myself about the perils of seeking a new beloved. Frankly, though, losing Ed has sharpened my desire for love and life and my sense of their impermanence. Our love gave me the courage and confidence to live wholly and freely and now that love is gone. Gone also is the "security" of living within it.

Since 2001 or so, Ed Epstein has slowly, and at times almost imperceptibly, been subject to a relentless reversal of his mental and emotional maturity, the insidious unfolding of what I know, by 2009, is early onset Alzheimer's disease. If you haven't known such a disease in your own life, it is hard to imagine how stealthily it approaches its victims and their families. Ed was torn away from me inch by inch and in the most confusing ways. Although most people would imagine there might have been a vivid scene in which his impairment was clearly revealed, in fact the erasure of his ability was slow, confounding, and provocative.

An imagined "classic scene" of him wandering out on a winter day or leaving the flame on the stove lit after cooking never occurred. Ed never wandered and he didn't cook. A few times he would forget to put the lid on the gas tank after he pumped gas, but that was rare enough not to stand out. His impairment was more insidious: He would be unable to put things into sequence, to make decisions, or to take initiative, but he covered all this up with his extraordinary verbal skills and personal warmth. Even now, I don't know how much he knew of his own impairment before it was conclusively diagnosed when the disease was quite advanced. For some time he and our friends thought I had become "just plain bossy," telling him what to do and how to do it. But I could feel something missing in Ed and I tried to compensate for it.

I recall a situation sometime in 2008 when he became incensed with me because I insisted I needed to make a tuna-salad sandwich for him. "I can make it myself!" he protested. Then he recited a clear verbal account from the first step (open the can of tuna) through the last step (spread the tuna salad on the bread slices). And so, I took out all the ingredients from the cupboards and set them in front of him. He could not begin. He could not see what came first, although he could say it. In his frustration, he broke down and cried. He could say the sequence, but he could not see the sequence in his mind's eye and move his body accordingly.

By the time I am flying back from South Africa, Ed's mind's eye has been blind for quite some time. He is cognitively and emotionally a very young child. I cherish and support him in his new life in a residential care center. We are divorced. I know conclusively that Ed has advanced Alzheimer's disease, diagnosed when he was 59 years old. I am also easily $70,000 in debt from credit cards he had taken out, then had forgotten to pay or lost. He had written another $57,000 in checks to himself from our joint account and spent some of that money on items I was never able to discover. We had no savings or investments for retirement and we had cashed out our life insurance policies to cover the immediate financial crisis.

The bottom has dropped out of everything that promised security in my life—marriage, finances, and any vestiges of control over my circumstances. One day in the summer of 2008, for example, I receive a letter from an eldercare lawyer who has reviewed our situation: He advises me to divorce Ed immediately (because of the liability I bear for Ed's extensive debts and his need for Medicaid), file for personal bankruptcy, apply for Medicaid for Ed, and sell our house. Decades of Buddhist practice have shaped me to accept and remain "fascinated" by whatever is inescapable: to watch carefully and precisely how the inescapable changes me. I am then, in a sense, prepared for this disaster. As my life slips out of my control, I try to remain as steady, curious, and engaged as possible. When I get this devastating news from the lawyer, I literally take a seat, breathe out, and say to myself, "Everything has changed."

Then I phone a dear friend of mine, a woman my age who is a Buddhist priest at a little Soto Zen temple up the road. I ask her if I can live at the temple if I need to. When she says, "Of course," I relax. As long as I have a place to live and can rent an office for my therapy practice, I don't need to be afraid. I must now simply pay close attention to what is changing and what I need to do, given these new demands on my fragile life. Later, I phone my accountant and she assures me that I should not sell my home just yet.

By the time I am flying back from Johannesburg, I live alone in my home on almost 600 uninhabited mountainous acres (I own 11 acres) in central Vermont. I am still practicing my profession of Jungian analysis and psychology on a full-time basis, uncertain about my future in most ways. I remain grateful to have a "precious human life" (as the Buddhists teach) even in the midst of the tragedy and adversity. Living outside a conventional story line, I notice, has also brought a whiff of exhilaration: Nothing is business-as-usual in my personal life anymore. Still, I wonder about my search for a new partner. Is there something about me that is restless and should be tamed instead of indulged? I have always felt peculiar. Now I feel peculiar in a whole new way, living on the margins of conventional life.

Even in my childhood, I was an introverted, anxious, and serious little person with lots of energy and a wide variety of interests that I pursued with abandon. My parents, who had both grown up in poor mining families in West Virginia and had to leave school by the age of 13, found it hard to understand and accept me. And, no wonder: My interests were so different from theirs and I was, in fact, strange in many ways. For instance, between the ages of 7 and 8, I became an elective mute. I stopped talking at home and school, and I also ate very little and didn't play with other kids. At that time, I was contemplating the meaning of "war"—that human beings willingly killed one another. My parents were themselves too often immersed in emotional warfare, fights in which they made threats of violence. I also saw other members of my family threaten and engage in violence. The prospect of people willingly killing one another just became too much for me to bear. I dove into my inner world where I had "contact" with named and unnamed spiritual forces. Eventually, I recognized in my childish way that my withdrawal was causing my parents and teachers a lot of suffering and I slowly came back to speech.

I was an only child (although I had a foster sister for 3 years), living just next door to my father's older brother who had five unruly children with whom I congregated on the long unsupervised summer days. Because we had the same last name and almost the same home address, there was a way in which I was included in their reckless and exciting ragtag clan and given a taste of a messy life that fell outside conventions. Nevertheless, I enjoyed solitude and was bookish and studious. At the local public library (about 4 miles from my home), I enthusiastically read all the "classics"—moving from one book to the next, alphabetically, along the shelves. Still, I was most at home in the woods and with my animals (we had dogs, cats, chickens, rabbits, and ducks) and in my 4-H garden projects. From the second grade on (after coming out of my mute phase), I had perfect grades at school and high scores on standardized tests. Eventually I became the co-valedictorian of my large high school class, graduating with straight As, while working a 20-hour-a-week job as a long-distance telephone operator during my senior year (bringing the paycheck home to my parents).

All this led to my feeling equally like an excellent student and a social outlier. Whereas in some people these two sides might blend smoothly together, in me they were in conflict. Even now I feel a kind of pressure to do my best to be a "leader" or "teacher" and influence the unfolding of consciousness and compassion in human life on earth. Ranged against this pressure to be engaged is a desire to be quiet, contemplative, and ensconced in the natural (not human) world. I am a mix of contrasting desires: to be spiritual and secular, to live a simple life and still be cool and worldly. I also want to see into the underlying reality of everything from the military (with which I worked in a leadership development program for college students) to spiritual enlightenment (whose practices I have become familiar with over decades). Sometimes I wonder whether there is something about my extreme individuality that leaves me feeling a peculiar need to be known and accepted by another.

And yet, decades of doing psychotherapy and psychoanalysis have persuaded me that everyone longs for a truly personal love. In my bones, I know this kind of love cannot be explained by reproductive drives, emotional magnetism, sexual desire, attachment bonds, or any other kind of biological need. We keep trying to explain love as brain science and the biology of hormones, but those versions omit the most mysterious aspects of being human, especially our drive to see ourselves in someone else's eyes and to know ourselves through someone else's meaning.

My earliest passionate love was for my mother. We were extremely close in my youngest years and I totally adored her. But she turned harshly against me after I went away to college and began to develop and succeed in ways that were unknown to her. My father, a factory worker, was no help because my interests were foreign to him, too. By the time I was 12 or so, I could see I was a bad match for my parents. There was an intellectual and emotional chasm between us. I didn't blame them or feel angry; I simply felt odd and tried to look normal. When my mother's apparently uncompli- cated love for me turned to a complicated hatred and never reversed, I was stunned and hurt. As I entered fully into adulthood, I simply accepted her attitude as beyond my ability to change, but it left me somewhat wary of getting close to another. I am very private and can still seem aloof with many people while I can also be very chatty and at ease when I am with trustworthy dear ones, but there was no one with whom I had more ease than Ed Epstein.

My love for Ed was emotional, intellectual, physical, and spiritual. Our friendship and our sexual attraction seemed inexhaustible: We both beamed when the other entered the room. Our pleasures were similar in relation to aesthetics, food, and culture. We loved to gossip and share secrets and our similar working-class backgrounds made us relaxed with each other socially.

When my husband lost his mind, he was healthy, hand- some, and vigorous. I was also healthy and enthusiastic about our life together as it seemed to be unfolding. Plan- ning your future and sleeping nightly with your best friend

and lover who is gradually becoming childish and irresponsible shocks and transforms you in some unique ways. In my
case, it started to awaken a new perspective on love. In the
way an illness can clarify a sense of being healthy or suffering can clarify freedom, Ed's Alzheimer's disease began to
illuminate the nature of love.

Feeling loved by Ed meant he took delight in our
daily contact, wanting to see and accept me just as I was.
He wanted to hear the details. Every day he held up a mirror and helped me see myself through his eyes. I did the
same for him. The reciprocal sharing of our lives enhanced
the colors and tones of daily life. Our love offered a way to
transcend our individual separateness and step out of our
self-enclosure and it was mutual/circular/reciprocal. Our
love required empathy, mindfulness, equanimity, emotional maturity, open communication, and truth-telling.
Those skills are eroded and eventually erased in people
with Alzheimer's disease. When I look back over the long
road I have traveled in learning how to love and in helping others love, I have learned most through the tragedy of
loving someone with premature dementia. Ed's capacity to
know me as a particular person and keep me in mind was
scrubbed away in the endless storms of neurons dying. We
do not usually include "knowledge" as a component of love,
but I can say definitively from my experience that knowing
your beloved as a particular person and holding him or her
in mind *is* a requirement. Otherwise, that individual seems
only to fill a role and feels used or disregarded.

Many aspects of Ed's warm demeanor remain even now

and encourage others' understandable, but painful, remarks about how much he "loves and adores" me. That is what people tend to say when they feel a warm affection between two people who have spent their lives together. For years now, though, I have come to see what is wrong with these ideas because Alzheimer's has eroded Ed's capacity to keep me in mind in my particularity. Looking from the outside at the two of us walking hand in hand down a country road near his residential care center, with our old dog hobbling along next to us, you might think, "I hope I can share a love like that when I am in the final years of my life." But now I know that much more than affection and care are required for love to be sustained and sustaining.

Though I minister to Ed's needs on an ongoing basis, bear witness to his changing life, and see him for extended visits at least twice a week, we have—of course—no partnership. Ed has a heartfelt connection to me, but he cannot ask me a personal question. He reaches out sweetly and tenderly for hugs and kisses and wants to caress me, but he cannot picture me driving home, he does not know if I am ill, and he cannot imagine anything about me that is separate from him.

Loving Ed has moved me to ask about love itself: What is it? Why is it so easy to idealize or sentimentalize or conflate it with romance, attachment bonds, and needs? Why is true love so hard to find, to practice, and to trust? True love requires being deeply and precisely known and then accepted—with our flaws. Known first and then accepted. But that acceptance must include an ongoing desire to see and know your beloved again and again, moment to moment, as she or he changes with the impermanence of life itself. Just as we come to know the world by trying to see it as it is, rather than how we want it to be, love invites us to discover the truth about another as a way of coming to know that person, ourselves, and ultimately the world.

But why do we look for a mirror in another's eyes where we can relax and study our own perplexity, pain, and confusion? Why is this relaxation always contingent on being certain that we are not simply being used to meet the other's needs or subtly controlled by the other's demands? Stretched out across three seats on the flight to London, I fade into a soft sleep and wake within the feverish grasp of a question: What is love, anyway?

THE PRESENT HEART

I.

Ed Epstein was my third husband. This fact might make you think I took marriage lightly, but just the opposite was true. I got married too quickly because I wanted to do the *right* thing. And, maybe more important, I didn't know how to evaluate the men who stepped forward and wanted to marry me. Marriage #1 and Marriage #2 were to men who were much older than me: They idealized me and needed me and I thought that meant they loved me. I am sympathetic to my younger self, as I have come to understand her, but she was clueless about choosing a partner and often confused about what she was looking for. As I look back now, I don't regret my "starter marriages." My growing up being what it was, I congratulate myself on doing as well as I did. It was hard to find a partner when I didn't know how to look for one, perhaps even harder because I confused being loved with being needed. I always felt my mother "loved" me when she mostly needed me for emotional comfort and sharing.

My first marriage took place in my senior year of college. I married a philosophy professor, 15 years older than me, who pursued me for a year with the conviction that he and I were meant for each other. I was Richard's third wife and became the mother of his second and third children as well as the stepmother for his first son. If I had had my eyes open, I might have wondered about these facts, but they seemed irrelevant at the time. We divorced when I was 27 years old and I moved away (with our two young children) to a distant city and began my graduate studies. Richard and I have remained friends over the years. I am also a friend of his second wife (the one before me) who is the mother of my stepson, my children's half brother. For most of my children's growing up, they had plenty of contact with their father. Grown up now, my children recognize how ill matched their parents are.

My second marriage, when I was 28, was to one of my graduate school professors, 11 years older than me, who pursued me for a year with the conviction that I was meant for him. Both of my first husbands were intelligent, articulate, and well educated. They had generous spirits and they wanted and needed me, but they were not interested in really getting to know me on a first-person basis. I filled up a place in them that had been empty and that was that. In the first 12 years of my adult life, in which I was mostly married (as a friend once said of me, I was "single for about 10 minutes"), I can now say I was unsure if the person I was sleeping next to in bed could even be called my "friend." My marriages, like most marriages back then, were not reciprocal or mutual. My husbands and I were not equals. As Jane Fonda has aptly put it, they wanted me to be in their stories, but they didn't want to be in mine.

I did not try to change them or rebel against them. As I had with my mother, I tried to adapt to the ways they needed me until I could no longer do so without losing my life force. With Ed Epstein, by contrast, my life force was enhanced and my being was increased. One of the extraordinary things about my relationship with Ed was that I met him before I had married either of these other men. On January 2, 1969, I took a plane from Cleveland, Ohio, to New York City where I was to rendezvous with Richard. He wanted to marry me, but I was unsure about my love for him. When I boarded the plane, I immediately spied in the row behind me what seemed to be an interracial gay couple: two men seated side by side with the black man's hand cozily placed on the white man's thigh. "That's interesting," I thought to myself, having never before seen such a couple. Turning around, I slyly stared through the space between the seats. Then the white guy suddenly popped up and sat down next to me. "Hi," he said. "My name is Eddie Epstein and I noticed you looking at me." Ed was tall, slender, and, it seemed to me, impossibly handsome. He looked directly at me with large liquid deep-brown eyes through long lashes that curled up. His manner was earnest and anxious and his thick black hair rippled down to his shoulders. He told me he was a theater student at New York University and was lonely and confused. He said that he wasn't gay but had brought home a gay friend from his program because he liked the guy and he wanted to shock his parents. He told me about his life and his difficulties in finding a relationship with a woman (something about there being so many gay men in the theater program and so few women?). Nothing like this had ever before happened to me! Ed was well-spoken, vulnerable, and seemingly open and honest. I still recall what it felt like to be looking straight into his face: It felt like we had known each other forever. The whole thing was exhilarating and frightening and confusing.

When he asked about me, I told him about Richard waiting for me at the Integral Yoga Society in uptown Manhattan. I told Ed that Richard had been pursuing me, wanting to marry me, but I was ambivalent. I also told Ed about the year I had just spent abroad in Europe and how it had changed my perspective on myself and my life.

When our plane landed, Ed asked me to have dinner with him. "Don't marry that man. He's too old for you." I had never before gone off with a stranger—and certainly not with someone who had a male companion—but there was something about Ed that seemed totally familiar and immediately trustworthy. His openness felt just like mine. I was 21 years old and a senior at Ohio University; Ed was 20 years old and a junior at New York University. I got into the taxi with him and his obviously angry friend (who jumped out during a red traffic-light stop in Manhattan) and we continued talking. After dinner we talked all night, and then, the next day, I called Richard to meet us for dinner in the Village. The three of us had an awkward, but friendly, dinner at a Chinese restaurant where Ed and Richard got exactly the same message in their fortune cookie—"You have a mutual friend." They had a laugh over that.

Although Ed had made a huge impact, and he wanted a long-distance relationship with me, I reluctantly said good-bye to him and chose to be with Richard. I felt Ed was too young and confused to provide the "stability" my life seemed to call out for (in fact, I was too young and con-fused). Later in 1969, I married Richard, who convinced me he would "provide security." In the interim between meeting Ed and marrying Richard, Ed and I talked many times by telephone and became friends. I invited Ed to my wedding. He made the long trek on a Greyhound bus from New York City to Athens, Ohio. He showed up after the wedding but was in time for the party. Ed seemed excited to see me, and he brought me the Judy Collins album that included the song "Pretty Polly." Even on the evening of my marriage to Richard, I had the strong feeling that Ed and I belonged together. When Richard and I divorced in 1974, I tried to find Ed. I called all the phone numbers I had for him, but none of them worked. In 1975, I got married again.

Then Ed stepped back into my world without my knowing it. He was a graduate student in a seminar I was teaching in the fall of 1981 at Bryn Mawr College where I was on the faculty of the Graduate School of Social Work and Social Research. Ed enrolled in it as a part of his mas-ters degree in clinical social work. It was a clinical semi-nar on counseling skills, and Ed and I sat across the table from each other for 90 minutes twice a week in class and sometimes we ran into each other outside of class, too. For 6 months, we did not recognize each other because repression was at work. Repression is an unconscious barrier against recognizing something you already know—something that would make you terribly anxious if you recognized it. Ed was now a balding middle-aged man with a beard, no longer slim. When we spoke to each other outside class, we often felt nervous (as we discovered later when we talked about it). Once he slipped on the ice in the parking lot and fell down hard on his side. I felt a shock run through me when I touched his arm to help him up. Although our appearances had changed a lot (not only was Ed different, I no longer had a hippie-style), repression played a bigger part in hiding our actual identities—who we were to each other.

On the morning of March 2, 1982, a dream got past my repression: In the dream, I am in bed with Ed as he was when I met him in 1969. I am startled to recognize that he is Eddie Epstein because I know I have an Ed Epstein in my class. I wake up and say to myself, "Could that be the student in my class?" Soothing myself—"I never forget a face; that couldn't be the same guy"—I go back to sleep. Once again, I have the same dream, but the man in bed with me is older. Again, I wake with anxiety and go back to sleep. The second time I go back to sleep, I dream of being in bed with my student!

Ed was scheduled to do a clinical presentation in my seminar—about an African-American family he was seeing, under supervision, in therapy about their son who was gay.

Of course, reading his case report contributed to lifting my repression. When Ed came by my office to pick up the video equipment, I asked him to step inside. "Last night I had a dream about a man I knew maybe 15 years ago. He was from New York City and his name was Eddie Epstein," I say hesitantly. Ed looks nervous. "I was a student in New York City around that time, but I don't remember you. There are a lot of people with the Epstein name." "I met this guy on an airplane flying from Cleveland, Ohio, to New York City in 1969." Ed looks more nervous. "Geez, that's odd, because I grew up in Cleveland, but I really don't remember you." "This Eddie Epstein was studying acting in New York," I say, narrowing my gaze to his eyes. "Man, I studied acting in New York City, but I really don't remember you!" "This Ed Epstein came to my wedding in Athens, Ohio, where I married Richard," I say with a dry mouth, feeling faint. "Oh my God! Polly, that was me!" We stare at each other. Lenses are shifting like tectonic plates inside me, bringing a new life into focus. "Oh, no!" I say silently to myself, "I will NOT tear my life apart again! I will not disrupt my children. NO. I don't care about love. NO!" Ed suggests we meet up later in the day to talk about what "has happened in our lives since 1969." Then we step right into the seminar where he stumbles awkwardly through his presentation.

My second marriage has already reached a point of conflict and disruption: I do not confide in my husband about any of my feelings or inner life. I often keep him at arm's length. I seek counsel from my friends, but I don't count my husband as a friend. We had married in St. Louis in 1975, and we were trying to build a family with our four young children in tow: ages 2, 3, 4, and 5 at the time of our union. His children stayed with us during the summers and other times when they could be away from their school in Washington, DC. My second husband offered Richard, my first husband, a job at the college where we worked, so Richard moved into a small house across the street from our modest two-story bungalow in a suburb of St. Louis. My children often ran through the neighborhood shouting "Daddy!" to different guys.

I entered serious long-term psychotherapy (eventually it became analysis) right around this time. I had had some psychotherapy during my first marriage also, but now I was beginning to see more clearly the nature of my unconscious dynamics. I try to speak haltingly to my husband about my insights, but they make no sense to him. I can tell that his initial idealization of me is turning into resentment. Our relationship begins to feel like a repeat of what happened between my mother and me.

I become a doctoral student in psychology at Washington University. When I graduate in 1980, I am offered a tenure–track teaching position at Bryn Mawr College, just outside Philadelphia. At the same time, my husband applies for a job in Chicago and we consider having a commuter marriage. We are not spending much time together as a couple, outside the time we spend as a whole family with the children, and we disagree about many things, especially spiritual and emotional issues. I am truly uncomfortable in my skin when we try to be intimate. All the same, we want to make our marriage work. Ultimately, he moves with me, and my children, and takes an administrative post working for the state of Pennsylvania. After arriving at Bryn Mawr College where we live in a house on campus, hardly a day passes that I am not nervous and unhappy. Settling into a whole new routine and taking on a new academic position while mothering young children means I am very stressed. My relationship with my husband is no comfort. Our disputes are serious, threatening, and disruptive. I continue in therapy by telephone and for a while he tries to find a therapist, but he does not find a good match.

This is the situation that Ed steps into when I remember him in my dream. Ed brings his current live-in partner (a woman 11 years his senior) to meet my husband and children. We try to have a dinner party, but there are a lot of suspicious glances going around the table. The next time we are slated to get together as a foursome (to "try to establish our friendship"), Ed phones to tell me he's broken up with his partner. "If I can't be with you," he says over the telephone, "then I want to find someone like you. You are exactly as I remember you from 1969 and you are the person I want to spend my life with." At first, I can't bear to hear what he's saying. I tell him that I am not available. Also, I point out that he needs to finish the academic year (he had about a month still) and graduate before we can even have another conversation. The whole situation feels crazily dangerous and simultaneously, entirely right.

In the summer of 1982, after his graduation, Ed and I begin having conversations about ourselves and our lives.

Keeping notes of my dreams and speaking to my therapist and my friends about my wrenching dilemma, I come to terms with the fact that Ed is the person I should have married in the first place. Mysteriously, we have been brought back together. One other significant event influences me: Katharine Hepburn speaks at Bryn Mawr College. To say I admire her is an understatement. I feel as though Hepburn is a major role model: Her independence, her modesty and understatement, her creativity, and her obvious vitality and courage always called to me, especially in those years. In an interview with her I attend at the college, she answers a question about her 30-year relationship with Spencer Tracy who remained married to someone else, and had additional extramarital affairs, during their entire relationship. Had she ever regretted it? "I have tried to live without regret," Hepburn replies firmly. "I loved Spencer deeply and well. We had a wonderful life together. I never regretted it for a moment." When I hear Katharine Hepburn say she lives without regret, I take that as a mantra. Knowing that I would deeply regret walking away from Ed, I decide to go through a second divorce. And so, in October 1982, I take the first steps to separate and divorce my second husband, a heart-wrenching loss for our whole family.

On January 13, 1985, after investing in a variety of psychotherapies for ourselves and our family, Ed and I marry at Pendle Hill, a Quaker retreat center in the suburbs of Philadelphia. Falling in love is no qualification for being in love. After we start living together and working with the angst and pain of a complex blended family, we have many quarrels and all-night dramas, looking at every aspect of our fears and fantasies about what would/could happen in the family and careers we are trying to build together. But as we move through these early years of transforming our passion into an abiding bond, I never stop trusting him or being attracted to him—and we never stop talking.

He and I engage in endless conversation and written correspondence (we'd write out our thoughts if we couldn't talk about a subject) about everything we want to know, say, or investigate with each other. We trust each other even to look into the unconscious hurts and themes that crippled us in our early lives. In these ways, we come to have a friendly knowledge (not an accusing "Do you know how you treat me like your mother?" kind of approach) of each other's unconscious dynamics and entanglements.

Though Ed came to have true affection and respect for my parents (and they, him), he sees how brutal my mother's envy and resentment had become in her relationship with me. He also witnesses the misery and violence of my father's mental illness, a borderline personality disorder that expressed complex serious trauma in my father's early life: When my father was 6, his father was murdered (for cheating at gambling), and when he was 10, his mother committed suicide. On many occasions, Ed protects me when we visit my parents (once or twice a year in their small working-class Florida community where they had retired). Ed's companionship on such a visit and our willingness to work together as a team (drawing on humor as well as our psychoanalytic ideas) transform tense and troubling encounters into scenes from a family sitcom. We enjoy even the difficulties.

It is similar visiting Ed's family: He has never felt truly known and often felt as though he had to embrace a persona (good-hearted, uninformed, naive simpleton) that was thrust upon him. His family requires a group identification in which everyone is submerged as an individual and Ed is not able to participate. He wants to be known for who he is instead of being "one of the Epstein boys." He feels like an outsider with his parents and his siblings. Visits with his family become "processing sessions" on our car trips back home. We talk for hours, bickering about what we'd witnessed, using the tools of our trade to deconstruct the emotionally troubling scenes, and finally coming around to some version of accepting our families with all their flaws and problems. But this "acceptance" includes knowing really and clearly how hurt and alienated each of us felt in growing up in our families—and how emotionally hard it is on us to visit now.

We are witnesses to each other in our emotional pain from past and present and we trust each other to go deeply into our own conflicts. Our ideas and ideals about our blended family, parenting, lovemaking, working together, and building our lives are never a smooth and easy fit; we often see things from different points of view. Ed has an inherently laid-back manner and I have an inherently straight-on directness. As much as our underlying spiritual and relational values are in sync, our styles are not. But we never tire of reviewing *everything* that requires review and we never stop making love.

At one point, before we married I believe, I turn to him when we are riding somewhere in the countryside and remark, "I didn't know it was possible to be so close and unguarded with another person." He agrees. Neither of us had ever experienced this kind of reciprocal love in which we felt free to express our individuality. And what is it—this "true love"? It is the means by which we each came to know and accept our selves and each other as individuals, as complete and completely recognizable human beings. We held up compassionate mirrors to each other that revealed even the disavowed, dark and aggressive or childish and regressive, tendencies next to the attractive, creative, and life-giving sources within us. Our fragile human lives were revealed in a light that made them intriguing, aesthetic, and profound between us.

The conditions in which Ed and I came to love each other are highly imperfect, even offensive to some: They were based on breaking up other relationships and choosing a partner who came from the Unknown—coming out of nowhere on an airplane, reappearing in a seminar, being identified in a dream. Only our closest friends originally "approved" of our union, if indeed they really did approve. Of course, in later years, as the richness of our relationship became evident to our friends and family and was witnessed even by strangers, we loved to tell the story of how we met and then lost and then found each other. The story became mythical although it was entirely factual. But when we were actually reunited, I was very afraid of my desire to be with Ed—its potential harm to my children and my second

husband and his children—but more afraid of living with
the regret of refusing a powerful offer that had twice
emerged from a mysterious source. I have never regretted
choosing Ed, not for a moment.

And this destiny continues still. Ed's deep acceptance
of his constrained new life—even with the emotional and
physical distance between us—brings a great comfort to
me. My close care for and witnessing of him bring an obvious comfort to him. Without fanfare or sentimentality, we
accept each other, just as we are, in a manner that lets us
be better people together than we would be apart. Some
might call this "unconditional love," but I call it "true love."
Although it is not immune to changes that are linked to
conditions, it is immune to the vicissitudes of conditions.
Our love has never been a prison in which we have lived
for any conventional reasons; instead it has been a space of
truth and vulnerability.

To give you a picture of what our relationship is like in 2012:
I drive about a hundred miles round-trip twice a week—at times
through snow and ice and other difficult road conditions—to
show up at the care center where Ed lives. Although the staff
makes sure he is washed and dressed before I arrive, telling
him I am on my way, he is always surprised to see me. "Oh,
Polly!" he says and sometimes adds, "Darling!" On some occasions, it seems he finds my sudden appearance uneventful—
his surprise sounds more like "Oh, it's you again"—as though
I'd been in the next room all along. At other times, he seems
shocked out of his mind and his hands and arms tremble and
his heart races. Whichever, he greets me with all his being. Ed

is still tall and nice-looking (except that his eyes are empty), weighing just over 200 pounds. He always loved stylish clothes and he still enjoys wearing warm colors and will (apparently, the staff tells me) wear only a couple of pairs of jeans because he feels the others of his many pairs of pants make him look "too old."

Ed cannot dress himself or go to the toilet alone. In the morning, an aide helps him shower and dress and brush his teeth. People from the staff check on him night and day and help him get to the toilet. Otherwise, he soils himself, and he is terribly distressed. His verbal skills and his ability to put on a persona (he was, of course, an actor in the first decade of adulthood) belie his confusion. Often he will phrase a few words—something like "Oh yes, let's get going!"—as though he is mastering what is going on. He cannot directly go to a table and sit down and eat. Someone has to guide him. He cannot directly get into the car or put on a shirt or jacket. He can still put on his cap and gloves and he's always pleased when he does. Ed is still able to carry a tune well and can, remarkably, sing many of the lyrics of songs he once knew. When he moved into the care center in early 2009, he could still recite some Shakespeare and poetry—lines that were etched into his mind from his early years in theater. Now those lines are gone. Sometimes we sing songs from his favorite songbook, *Rise Up Singing!* He prefers the "old chestnuts" (as he calls them): "I've Been Working on the Railroad" and "You Are My Sunshine" and a few Christmas songs (that have year-round appeal for him). He and I are able to sing together "Unchained

Melody" and "Try to Remember" even if we cannot get all the words and lines. He carries a tune better than I do and sometimes he complains if I get off-key, saying, "Let me do it alone!"

His care center is located in East Craftsbury, Vermont, in gorgeous countryside, on a country road looking out at a church, some fields and trees, and cows (when the weather permits). There are 23 residents and 24 staff and his room is delightful because I had it painted (one accent wall and the door) to replicate the colors of our living room. He has lovely wall art and a flat-screen TV (which is completely disconnected from the cable hookup because he cannot use it) and lots of music boxes that he cannot wind up (but loves me to wind). He is regarded as one of the "stars" of his care center because he is generally the youngest man, one of the warmest and most emotionally expressive residents, and definitely the most handsome. When he first moved there, he could still perform parts of favorite plays and the activities director made sure he had opportunities to do so. He still loves to hear poetry read to him and other residents recall when he could recite lines from memory.

Ed is usually vibrant and happy when I am around. Often he laughs constantly. On a recent family visit with him, my son remarked, "Ed is just a laughing Buddha now! Nothing upsets him." When I say, as I do repeatedly, "I love you so much, Ed," he usually replies, "I know." Sometimes he says, "I love you, too." From past conversations, I know that Ed wishes me well in my life and does not expect me to sit at home, emotionally or psychologically shut down. He has told me as much. I feel completely connected to Ed's spirit; he has been liberated through this disease in some very important ways. Without minimizing the tragedy of Ed's losing his mind, he has also been freed from the nervous self-consciousness and relentless feelings of inadequacy that plagued him through all the years he was well. He has now forgotten how to feel inadequate. When Ed and I are together, I feel little sadness and no regret. Instead, our love—as it is—feels very freeing.

In our earliest decades, the mirrors Ed and I held up to each other especially revealed our creative strengths and potentials, as we encouraged each other to become better therapists, to get more education or training, and to step into new roles. As embarrassing as it sometimes seems to me now, Ed and I began to work together as couples therapists in 1983, just a year after we re-met and before we married! He had a background in psychodrama and socio-drama: forms of dramatic role-playing and group therapy that forged the therapeutic roles of an "alter ego" and "audience," both of which we used in our model. I had been teaching and supervising family therapy and psychoanalytic object relations therapy: methods that look at the unconscious dynamics in couples and families.

Along the way, we became acquainted with Structural Family Therapy, developed by Salvador Minuchin and practiced at the Child Guidance Clinic of Philadelphia in the 1980s. In the 1980s, I finished my training to be a Jungian psychoanalyst and began to write books, especially about women's development—bringing a feminist orientation to depth psychotherapy. Structural Family Therapy unintentionally, but predictably, encouraged a sexist approach to a woman's role in the family and the couple relationship as it tried to "recentralize" the father. Ed and I both witnessed some disastrous unintended consequences of this form of therapy for mothers and their children.

In a flash of intuition, one day when I was out with Ed somewhere, I realized that he and I could put together a new form of dyadic (two therapists in the room) psychotherapy for couples that could integrate theories of unconscious relational functions, new insights of feminism and sex-role equality, along with some psychodrama techniques and Jungian theories of mythic and symbolic themes. I saw this as a way of opposing sexism in Structural Family Therapy and some other forms of family therapy; instead of simply criticizing the sexist therapies, we could start something new. As I write this now, it sounds ridiculously ambitious and optimistic and yet, it worked. One day, I casually say to Ed, "We could do couples therapy together and come up with a new model that integrates our different skills." Characteristically, he replies, "Who would want to come to see us? I don't know a thing about couples therapy." And so it goes. After hashing through the particulars, we draw up a model of how our sessions might look, what their goals would be, and we begin to offer couples therapy at a very low fee while we develop our capacity to work together as a team.

In the early days, Ed and I spent at least 2 hours processing every hour of therapy we did together! Also, we found that the couples we saw stirred up plenty of unfinished business between us. All the same, by 1984, I publish a book (my first book) entitled *Hags and Heroes: A Feminist Approach to Jungian Psychotherapy with Couples.* The book is grounded in a folktale from the Middle Ages called "Sir Gawain and the Lady Ragnell"—a story I had studied in my senior year in college. Ed memorizes the story and loves to tell it in a dramatic form at the workshops and seminars we give to train therapists in our method. The second half of the book is a manual for doing what we call "Dialogue Therapy," which integrates all of the moving parts I had imagined it would.

Ed and I then begin to specialize in doing, teaching, and supervising Dialogue Therapy. We teach other therapists how to do it and present programs at national conferences, trainings, and videotape demonstrations of it and its principles. Dialogue Therapy—a structured short-term form of dyadic psychodynamic psychotherapy for couples—is highly effective when it is a good match with a particular couple. Ed and I continue to work together doing and supervising it until he is unable to keep up in the sessions. We teach many other therapist teams to use it and feel very proud of how many couples are helped to find greater emotional ease and freedom in their lives together. For more than a decade, Dialogue Therapy provides the greatest opportunity for my growth as a therapist because it quickly shows the presiding therapists how symbiotic entanglements hinder couples' intimacy. The couple and the therapists work on new skills of differentiation and acceptance to heal those entanglements. A second book on couples and Dialogue Therapy is published in 1993: *You're Not What I Expected: Love After the*

Romance Has Ended. I wrote it from the years of practicing, teaching, and supervising that Ed and I did together.

After I finished some of the initial promotion for this book and signed a contract for my next book, Ed and I move to Burlington, Vermont, in 1994 to begin a new life. For the first time since we became a couple, we separate our clinical practices, though we continue to do, teach, and supervise Dialogue Therapy together. In Philadelphia, Ed often complained that I had "supervisory" power over him in our joint practice because I had a doctorate and was "president" of our psychological corporation and he had a masters in social work and could not hold the position of president. I could see how this inequality provoked both of us. Ed's work habits often made me nervous because he rarely kept up with details and forms—of which there were many. Ed always had problems with sequencing, initiative-taking, and decision-making—some of the executive functions that are wholly undermined by Alzheimer's. As I have reflected back on some of Ed's habits of mind and behavioral struggles, I have come to believe that Ed suffered some neural condition that predisposed him to the disease. It was as though he had an organic weakness around which his neuronal functioning eventually collapsed.

Once Ed and I become separate business entities, working in our own settings, I can see both Ed's strengths and weaknesses more objectively. His strengths are clearly his personal warmth, his empathy, and his deep acceptance of human frailties. He has an unerring ability to put people at ease and to offer any feedback or challenge so deftly and softly that others sign on to it almost immediately, feeling they have probably come up with the idea themselves. Since Ed has been ill, many former patients of his have reached out to me to say how deeply transformative and helpful their therapy with him had been. He helped many and never gave up on anyone because they ran out of funds or failed in some other way.

But Ed's disorganization and lack of efficient record keeping interfered with his own feelings of confidence. He often portrayed himself to colleagues and to me as being on the verge of a nervous breakdown—unable to stay on top of anything that demanded regular discipline and management. He depended on me to help him with record keeping, exercise, meditation, and his calendar. Ed was unhappy with himself for these shortcomings, but I came to accept them as part of our relationship. I also eventually accepted that, in social situations, Ed would often ask others for help as though he couldn't handle his life; he'd ask for help with diet, finances, and health concerns, but he would not follow through on the advice he was given.

In 1995, I made a trip to Asia and was away from home for almost 5 weeks. This is a painful separation for the two of us because telephone contact (there is no e-mail) is difficult and I can write only postcards or short notes to Ed; my schedule is busy with lectures in Japan and visiting my daughter who is in the Peace Corps in Thailand. When I return to Vermont, Ed tells me he has started taking an antidepressant and Ritalin. I am stunned. We take a long walk (maybe 10 miles or so) along Lake Champlain to review what Ed's experience has been while I was gone. Through tears and shouting and then stepping back and asking questions, we come to a shared perspective that Ed has "an unhappiness within him" and that "he is entitled to it." He believes I want him to be happy in a way he cannot achieve. I always hoped Ed would find an enduring happiness and be able to enjoy the rich pleasures of our amazing life; he is very happy with me—he says our marriage is the "best thing" he's ever done—but he is relentlessly unhappy with himself and that unhappiness spills over into how he feels about his life. Ed has a core feeling of inferiority and shame that has haunted him since childhood. In that fateful conversation on the shores of Lake Champlain, Ed and I come to an agreement that ironically gave us comfort: He has a right to his own unhappiness, feeling of inferiority, and shame. I will never again try to encourage him to "do something" about these states. They are his, not mine.

Tragically and paradoxically, only Alzheimer's has relieved Ed of his deep unhappiness; years of psychotherapy and meditation couldn't do it. Ed and I have repeatedly embraced the understanding that his disease has a karmic meaning. My entire relationship with Ed has a karmic feel to it. Meeting Ed in 1969 was remarkable. Finding him in 1982 was magic. I had been looking for him for more than a decade—not every day or everywhere, but he had generally been in my rearview mirror. And then, weirdly, he showed up across the table in my seminar at Bryn Mawr College.

When Ed reappeared in my life, I was stunned and shocked. I felt as though the universe had arranged this and that I was subject to impersonal forces that exist far outside my knowledge and control. I was destabilized, afraid, excited, and amazed by the strength of repression (never again did I question whether it was possible to repress something that had really happened) and the presence of mystery in my life. Then, after 20 years of breaking open each other's hearts through our extraordinary partnership, impersonal forces strike us again, rearranging us, just as we are settling down to live out our dreams on the side of a mountain in Vermont. This time, those forces take the form of harsh and enlightening lessons from Alzheimer's disease.

2.

Starting around 2001 when Ed was 53 years old, he began to show perplexing behaviors in his everyday life. At first, I noticed he was often bored or indifferent in social gatherings. His warm demeanor—a hallmark of his personality—would belie his indifference, but he would stay well in the background of conversations, rarely speaking, and sometimes would actually fall asleep while another person was talking with him, especially after dinner. He missed appointments, forgot to pay bills, and worried day and night about what seemed to be trivial details of his work. Sometimes he spent hours (even staying overnight in his office) filling out forms for his job as a high school social worker or later as a public mental health counselor. He had overwhelming problems with short-term memory—keeping track of what he was supposed to be doing—as well as poor judgment about spending and finances. He eventually neglected every aspect of our relationship and his roles around the house. In his anxiety, he would even forget to say "Good morning!" He was so distracted about completing his professional tasks that he wouldn't eat with me, talk to me, or make any social plans.

By the summer of 2006, almost everything I had known and wanted in my personal life was somehow falling apart. My marriage, my financial stability, and my trust in Ed were becoming bizarrely disrupted in ways that were hard to acknowledge and impossible to explain. My children and other family members begin to back away when they see I am facing what seems to be a bottomless pit of financial and emotional disasters. The financial collapse and the inevitable obfuscation connected to Alzheimer's disease naturally make it hard for others to believe I know what I am doing. I myself can barely embrace the cascade of losses even with my spiritual commitment to do so. All vestiges of conventional well-being and security—except my capacity to earn a living—have been destroyed. Many who know me well begin to lose confidence in my decision-making. When I try to explain my "Zen" attitude (remaining interested and engaged with my life, step by step, exactly as it emerges) few find it convincing as a long-term plan.

A pivotal event had taken place during May 2006: a Buddhist conference-retreat in Kyoto, Japan. During the event, it became obvious that Ed was, in fact, somehow losing his mind. This was a trip Ed did not want to make. As I look back now, I realize that he was panicked about his functioning (he had lost two jobs by then because he couldn't complete the administrative tasks). Ed knew that he was not able to keep up with others, but he didn't want to acknowledge this fully to me or even to himself. Almost as soon as we arrived in Japan, Ed came down with a bad sore throat and high fever that drew away whatever resources he had available to cover his impairment in social situations. He could not sequence his thoughts or figure out what was going on around him.

Ed's impairment was obvious and many people were made uncomfortable by it. I was one of the organizers of the event: a Zen retreat and conference in which Europeans, Americans, and Japanese came together to meditate and talk about the commonalities and differences between Zen Buddhism and depth psychotherapy. Ed mostly stayed in our hotel room, and conference attendees—many of whom had known Ed personally from an earlier conference in Japan—wondered why. Eventually a friend and I took Ed to the hospital (because of his high fever) where he was put on IV antibiotics for an afternoon. Then he was released into my care on oral medicine. We left Kyoto the next day to attend a 4-day retreat at a Zen monastery in northern Japan. The Japanese doctor had assumed a Zen retreat would not make too many demands on Ed, but his inability to carry out instructions in ceremonies and complete the tasks that he was assigned was apparent to everyone.

After the retreat, feeling afraid and exhausted by what I had witnessed, I had a conversation with a colleague from South Africa on the bus ride back to Kyoto. On that ride,

Deon—a man around my age—spoke to me passionately about caring for his wife who had died just 2 years earlier of breast cancer. Working through his loss and discovering a new identity were among the reasons he had come on this trip. I was impressed by his willingness to speak transparently about the stress, sadness, and inherent pleasures of caring for the dying. At the conclusion of the conference, I said good-bye to my new friend with a group of others who waved him off as he left on a bus.

When I returned home after the retreat I began to look closely into our bank accounts and finances (which Ed had always managed) and to uncover egregious errors and oversights. Seeing this financial evidence in the light of what I had witnessed in Japan, I began to suspect that something was seriously wrong with Ed's mind although I couldn't allow myself to express this idea to anyone but my closest friends.

During this time, I also began to read expert advice about caring for those who have dementia: Caregivers should not correct or "demand reality" from those who cannot keep up with their context. I try to do this, but often feel stumped in determining what Ed wants or needs without demanding some reality. I repeat questions about what he would like to eat or where he is going. I recall saying, on several occasions, something like "For the thirty-sixth time, I am trying to find out . . ." and then feeling ashamed when Ed looks crushed and confused. I draw on my meditation practice to simply feel my feelings without a narrative and then return to ask Ed patiently (mostly patiently) my questions without such exasperation. I tell myself to "take things one step at a time" and that "we really don't know what is happening to Ed."

I also take up the hunt for miracle cures. I look into homeopathy, herbal treatments, Brain Gym, massage, and shamanism. For each one of these, I work hard to find the "best" and "most scientific" approach. It takes energy and courage from both Ed and me to traipse around from healer to healer. Finally, a Vietnamese herbal doctor—Dr. Quang Van Nguyen who practices in Bennington, Vermont— looks me in the eye one afternoon when Ed and I are sitting across from him, and he says something like "His brain no good. Don't go to no more doctors. No more money." We still don't have a diagnosis. Though I am grateful for Dr. Quang's honesty, I remain open to miracle cures.

Sleeping with Ed poses a problem for me. I can "feel" into his mind when his head is on the pillow next to me; at times, it seems that my dreams are drawn into his dreaming mind. I am restless in my sleep in some bizarre ways and have strange dreams in which Ed is taking apart our house or destroying what we have built. At some point, Ed can no longer recall his night dreams. In the absence of dreams, his night sleep feels totally dead. This is sad for both of us. Is he repressing his dreams or forgetting what has happened in them or both? Soon after this, I feel a kind of deadness in my sleep as well. I cannot recall my dreams. I make a decision to sleep in a separate bed.

Once I am sleeping alone, my morning meditation and dreams often reveal—in precise and practical ways—how to respond to various crises that are facing me. "Call this lawyer, make an appointment to see this doctor, check with this friend or this service." These directives are startling because they are precise, wise, and correct. I come to trust that a deep mind is awake within me. It knows the details of what I need to do even though I don't know them. If I can stay in touch with this deep mind, I will be okay: I will know how to deal with my circumstances. Although this development seems extraordinary—beyond anything I could have imagined—it also seems familiar. Even in my childhood I felt the presence of a reality beyond the visible world.

After I discover our financial ruin and begin to get medical help for Ed, I am working 35 to 40 hours per week doing Jungian analysis, psychotherapy, and clinical supervision, while managing Ed's daily care. I also have to finish writing a book that is contracted to come out in 2008. I have no choice about my long work hours; we need every penny I make. And so, I practice encountering what emerges moment by moment with a gentle matter-of-fact acceptance (an attitude of "and now there is this and this and this"). Doing psychotherapy with others also provides relief for me. During therapy sessions, I can live in someone else's life.

In early January 2008, I notify our friends about the severity of Ed's symptoms and the fact that he has to surrender his license to practice clinical social work and is formally retiring. I send out an e-mail to our Buddhist community e-mail list (Deon is on that list) that begins, "This is a difficult note to write, but I've wanted you to know—and some of you already know—that Ed is suffering from a serious memory impairment that has led to some cognitive impairment as well. This condition has been developing slowly over the years but has taken a definite turn for the worse over the past 6 months or so." The e-mail concludes, "Ed is retiring. He'll be applying for disability and doing various jobs around our place. Of course, this has been tremendously difficult for him (demoralizing and anxiety-making) and for me (worrying and dispiriting)."

The following day, my South African friend Deon responds: "I can only imagine how anxious and uncertain you must feel about the time ahead. I just wonder what qualities it will take to manage in the best ways you can. I remember with my late wife, that during the last years of her illness, my time-frame started moving from getting through week by week, to day by day, to hour by hour." His interested and engaged tone immediately warms my heart. I am lonely and need a little heartwarming.

Soon after that first e-mail exchange, Deon and I begin an e-mail correspondence that consists of my sharing my personal trials and reflections and his sharing his reminisces about his wife's dying. This is how we begin to get to know each other although we already have plenty in common. As our e-mails get more frequent and are accompanied by phone conversations, we offer ideas and views about each other's lives. Not long after that I begin to feel I am falling in love with a virtual stranger who lives 8,000 miles away!

I was shocked at the intensity of my feelings. My

interlocutor was providing something in his empathic and mindful witnessing that increased my vitality and interest in my everyday life. Perhaps because there was no physical contact between us, I could see how the horizons of love and desire take shape from the reciprocal revealing of our selves—as particular individuals. Deon wasn't always perfectly attuned, but he asked me questions with an open heart. "What was that like? How did it affect you?" And as he mirrored my ideas and experiences back to me in a new light, their meanings opened up. I did the same for him and I was also not perfectly attuned, but we soon began to talk about those imperfections and our conversations got more interesting and lively. Gradually, we both came to depend on these exchanges for friendship and support. Of course, we were meeting on the ground of loss and change. Each of us had experienced things that were hard to speak about in ordinary conversation.

Over several months, Deon and I easily fall into intoxicating Skype conversations about our lives, our families, and our ideas. Like me, he is a Jungian psychologist. Like me, he has been married a couple of times and is very close to his family, including his grown daughter, and even has a friendly relationship with his daughter's mother. Like me, he grew up with hardship and became resilient. He'd lost his second wife to breast cancer, and he'd learned a lot in tending her through her dying. His politics are attractively progressive and his values are deeply humanitarian. He's been on many Buddhist retreats and uses those practices in his everyday life.

When I go to visit him in South Africa, I believe I am in love with Deon. We have been speaking to each other regularly on Skype and we have met in person several times before this trip. On the return trip, however, I notice that I have become acutely aware of a fact I had been avoiding: that we come from very different cultures. Deon's native language is not English, but Afrikaans. After meeting his mother, sisters, brother, daughter, and close friends, I have come to feel more like a stranger when I look into his eyes. A visceral difference of meaning has become palpable and I begin to wonder if the love I have promised is rooted in idealization and desire rather than reality. And as it happens, our relationship ends in June 2010, almost 3 years ago as I write this.

We parted as friends and remain so. The reality of having any kind of embodied relationship with Deon was impossible. I could never leave Ed. My devotion to him is absolute. Deon did not want to move to Vermont and leave South Africa, his family home for more than two generations. Deon and I continue to be deeply grateful for the bond that took shape around our losses. In addition to our friendship, almost 2,000 e-mails remain from my correspondence with him in 2008. These e-mails give precise details and insights on my daily life from that time. I will include excerpts (in italics) from my side of the correspondence in order to clarify what it was like to move from the chaos of not knowing what was happening to knowing that Ed's mental maturity had been permanently lost.

April 8, 2008

I awoke during the night and involuntarily mulled over the problem of what has been missing in the last 5 years of our relationship. Really, it's been the lack of witnessing that has been so hard. Ed rarely knows where I am, what I'm doing, what is going on in my physical or mental being. Ed is oblivious of me unless he needs me. Or, to put it more accurately, he just takes me for granted as a support and that is VERY hard because it is happening in addition to the enormous draw he has made on my financial and emotional resources. It's not just that Ed forgets my birthday, he forgets that I have a birthday!

He'll spend the better part of an hour trying to recall the name of a client of his, but he never asks me a question or shows any interest in what I have been doing. When we sat down to lunch today, he said suddenly, "Do you know what's on my mind?" and I replied in what I thought sounded like a humorous tone, "Well, I'm sure it's got nothing to do with me." That threw Ed and he said, "Yes, I do think about you." But then he couldn't go further; he couldn't recall what he had intended to say. And I said, "I bet you were trying to remember the name of your client" and Ed replied, "Yes! That's it." This feels like nonsense going back and forth between us as though we are trying to tune in to a faint channel that would allow us still to feel a connection and a confidence about being seen and known by each other.

For about 3 years before I moved Ed into residential care in early 2009, while he was still living at home, he frequently did something common to Alzheimer's sufferers: He imitates or piggybacks on what I say or do. This close tracking can create a lot of annoyance in me. When possible, I draw on my meditation practice to lighten my burden with humor or direct awareness—perceiving my feelings simply as body sensations and just "hearing" the commentary in my mind. One of the meditation practices I do is called *vipassana*, which means "seeing things as they really are" or "seeing into things with clarity and precision." Applying it allows me to study my responses by feeling and hearing and seeing them without adding a lot of narrative (like "Oh my God, I can't stand this one more minute!"). I can readily see how desperate Ed is to appear "normal" and how little freedom he has to be spontaneous. My heart often goes out to him even if I have feelings of annoyance.

I need help in taking care of Ed when I am working and when I am away from home. As I reach out to others, there are basically two kinds of responses. First, there is the rare response of real help: someone who listens closely, hears what is needed, and does exactly that. My longtime friend Heidi, for instance, came to stay with Ed several times when I went away. She did so with grace, humor, and generosity and she seemed to enjoy her stay. Heidi rarely complained and she sometimes sat with me, especially in the first couple of years, and listened to me trying to imagine a future. She knew my financial situation and she empathized with the demand it made on my time and energy without expressing any advice or judgments. Heidi was my college roommate and we had been close witnesses to each other's lives for almost 4 decades. When I moved Ed into residential care, Heidi stayed with me for 2 weeks. While I did my regular therapy hours, she sorted through Ed's clothes and papers. She threw things away, donated others, and got his belongings ready for the move. I cannot imagine I could have made this move without her help. Heidi's grace and generosity are unforgettable.

Jill, a friend from my Buddhist community, took Ed into her home while I was on retreat and stayed with him when I had to travel for my work and he suddenly needed a hospital procedure to repair a hernia. She was very supportive, lighthearted, and helpful. Still another friend from my Buddhist community, Margery, was very dear in caring for Ed when I was away and then joined me for a couple of hilariously sweet dinners. My son, Colin, and his wife, Melissa, came at crucial times to help with Ed and to assist me with his move to the care center. They have continued to visit Ed regularly, without question or encouragement from me.

The second kind of response to reaching out—ordinary and expectable, I came to see—is one in which the other person intends to be supportive or helpful but offers an opinion or advice that has precisely the opposite effect. In such cases, an opinion is typically offered instead of help. This kind of interaction intensifies the pain of what is missing: a way to relax and be oneself in another's presence. For example, a friend who was receiving a fee to provide care for

Ed after he had gone on disability, sits me down one evening, after I have been working 10 hours in my therapy office, and says, "I don't mean to pry, but I can tell your husband would benefit from having someone read to him. He loves this when I do it and I wonder if you could find some time to do it with him." Her tone implies, "If you could *only* find time in your busy schedule." Instead of diving across the room and strangling her, which is what I feel like doing, I reply in what I hope sounds like a calm voice, "I have known Ed since 1969. I know him well. He adores poetry and reading out loud. He and I have read together for years, and so, I wonder why you think I need your advice about this right now." She says, "I just thought you would want to know."

Such unintentionally disrespectful remarks feel to me like "micro-aggressions"—a term from studies of bias and racism that names the zingers meant to fall beneath our radar. I think all caregivers are sensitive to these micro-aggressions, but perhaps I had an extra dose of sensitivity because at the tender age of 7 years I saw, in my childish way, how people are motivated to hurt one another without recognizing their destructive aims. In my adult life, of course, I have studied and applied many psychoanalytic theories about envy, competition, and self-protection in our unconscious intentions toward one another. We are all self-protective and when we encounter another's suffering or pain, we may just automatically shield ourselves.

Over decades, I had heard about abandonment by friends and social alienation in the face of personal loss. Psychotherapy clients who had suffered difficult illnesses or accidents or had lost a spouse or a child typically told a story of being abandoned by friends and family in the midst of their loss. And so, it is no surprise when many turn away from me. Those under siege usually find this abandonment to be a terrible affront. As friends and family members fail to call or reach out to me, I determine not to take it personally or to react angrily. In certain ways, I feel tentatively well equipped to pay attention and be unafraid of what is unfolding.

Perplexity and uncertainty are my constant companions and I welcome them, as much as I can. I determine not to fashion a story line in which I was the victim or at fault for what was happening. Still, I often feel painfully set apart. I listen obsessively to Bob Dylan sing about disappointments and failures of loyalty and empathy. Hearing those facts plainly stated in his lyrics makes them easier to digest. As friends and family stop calling I say to myself, "Why shouldn't they back away? If they feel into my experience it might be painful for them, too."

My meditation practice has taught me both the means and the value of embracing my immediate experience for what it teaches and to accept change—even unwelcome change—as the fundamental ground of my life. This doesn't mean I am passive or uninvolved in changing what I can change, but simply that I am poised to accept and learn directly from conditions that are not under my control. Paying close attention to painful and unwanted life events opens doors to insight into the nature of the reality in which we are embedded.

As long as I don't deny my feelings but allow them to emerge into my body-mind and then to pass away, I can investigate with a gentle awareness what my life is now presenting me. I can see from the very start that my profound losses are also an opportunity. I am being tested by my life in my capacity to engage with circumstances that go against my own desires and fall fully outside of my will. To sharpen my awareness, I increase my daily meditation practice to an hour each morning and also attend several important meditation retreats even though this means I am away from Ed. I rise between 4:30 and 5:00 a.m. in order to meditate and record my dreams.

Dealing directly with Ed—his being and spirit—is a powerful transformative experience for me and for others. His many years of Buddhist practice assist him in accepting his disease. He even finds surprising meaning, insights he comes up with himself. For example, he begins to see "karmic" lessons in his cognitive impairments: "I have been too ego-oriented all these years," he remarks, "always comparing myself to others and feeling like I was inferior. I am forgetting to do that now!" In the summer of 2008, I spend hours talking with Ed, sometimes not knowing whether he understands what I say. It hardly matters because it is often easier to speak with him than to try to talk to others who regularly misunderstand me. From time to time, Ed shows clarity and generosity that come from a mysterious source. One day after neuropsychology tests confirmed his serious impairments, but before we have a diagnosis, Ed and I are swimming at our favorite pond. While swimming he says,

"I feel so sad about everything I am losing. I am losing my mind. I am losing our relationship." I say, "You are losing your mind, but you will never lose our relationship. We have a really deep love." He replies, "I know everything will be fine. This illness is making me more spiritual."

November 17, 2008

Ed was really scared in that cavernous waiting area for neurology patients at Dartmouth-Hitchcock hospital. He clung to me in the waiting room. When we were called into Dr. Coffey's office, he greeted us with the question "How's Ed doing?"—a question I felt was increasingly impossible to answer. Ed generally didn't answer. The doctor then said almost cheerily, "Well, we have a clear picture of what's been going on."

First, he handed me a printed report. "Findings: Markedly diminished metabolic activity in both frontal, temporal, and parietal lobes, relatively greater and symmetric metabolic uptake in both motor strips and visual cortices. Impression: Markedly diminished diffuse, bilateral activity frontal, parietal, and temporal lobes consistent with advanced Alzheimer's-type dementia." I was shocked to read the words—"advanced Alzheimer's-type dementia."

Dr. Coffey addressed us candidly. "Your condition may have begun with fronto-temporal dementia," he said, "but it has progressed rapidly and now you have an advanced Alzheimer's-type dementia." He was surprised. He'd had no idea Ed was "so progressed." Then Dr. Coffey put up a hologram of Ed's brain on the large computer screen. It was a very dire picture. I watched Ed wince; he was obviously terrified and humiliated by this picture of his brain. Dr. Coffey commented how it was "amazing" to be able to see the whole brain and to have a "conclusive diagnosis." We stared at a three-dimensional picture of Ed's brain floating in black space. There were great gaping black holes in the right frontal, parietal, and temporal lobes. Almost all of his "lights" (metabolic activity) were out, but Dr. Coffey pointed out that the left rear of Ed's cortex was still "lit up." This is where language functions reside. "Your high verbal functioning gives the impression that you are doing better than you are," the doctor said, apparently to comfort us for having been fooled about the extent of Ed's diminishment.

Then Dr. Coffey said emphatically, "Ed must stop driving." Up until that moment, I couldn't imagine stopping him from tooling around in his old black pickup truck. He didn't drive much and he went painfully slowly up the road to Montpelier from our house. But now Dr. Coffey reminded me that I was Ed's power of attorney and I would be directly responsible if Ed hurt anyone or damaged property. Dr. Coffey also suggested that I "look into a residential care facility. You won't be able to handle Ed's care alone." No one had said this to me previously. In fact, almost all our family and friends seemed to think that I could handle his care if I just got a few "social workers" to come in. Dr. Coffey concluded our meeting saying, "The good news is that you don't have to come back here and take any more tests. We know what is wrong now."

Ed and I stumbled out of the hospital into the parking

lot holding hands and crying. I was simultaneously terrified
and relieved. Now I knew what had been happening to him
and me over the past 5 or more years as he had changed so
dramatically. It wasn't a matter of "forgiving" Ed for the
unbelievable difficulties he'd caused. It was more a matter
of becoming conscious. I could still love him, but our rela-
tionship was no longer mutual and equal. It could never
be that again. Nothing could fix it. Everything was clear.

When friends encounter Ed's open-heartedness to the
changes brought about by his illness, they want to talk about
the effects he has on them. Although I want to hear what
they think and feel when they are with him, I also want to
avoid those hurtful micro-aggressions that may come with
others' opinions and views. I want to protect myself from
conventional ideals and stereotypes about love and spousal
bonds because I now find them offensive—"Isn't it amazing
how much Ed still adores you!"—or trivializing—"You need
to take a step back now and experience your own grief and
take care of yourself."

These quick formulations are distasteful and wrong.
It's as though these ideas are small boxes into which large
and mysterious contents are being shoved. I recall now how
Dan Gottlieb, a friend and radio talk show host whom I
interviewed for my book *The Resilient Spirit*, felt about
people remarking on his quadriplegia—the result of an
accident when he was 28 years old, 2 decades earlier then.
People would say things like "Isn't it great that you can still
raise your arms!" "No," Dan said to me, "it's not great. It's

a tragedy that I can use only a few muscles in my body."
When Dan first came home from the hospital after his accident and first surgery, he appreciated his young daughter
saying, "I hate you because you ruined my life!" "She was
speaking to me honestly," Dan remarked, "and that was a
relief." Too often I feel as though I cannot speak honestly
to my friends because they have no possibility of receiving
the complex mix of pain, sorrow, and excitement I feel. I
am both sorrowful and extra-open—feeling almost newly
minted in this world.

Some friends and family suggest I join a support group
for spouses of Alzheimer's patients, but I prefer not to. I
don't want to hear the bitterness and hurt expressed about
their abandonment by friends and family members. I don't
want to feel the hopeless drying up of caregivers' life energies. I don't want to be swept up into blame or fear or shame
or further alienation. And yet, I am gratefully aware of how
helping others and hearing their life stories helps me every
day in my therapy office. I don't want to expose my own
story because I am trying to see it freshly. I don't want to
have a model or narrative imposed on it.

On some public occasions—talks and presentations—
when it seems potentially of use to others, I mention that
my husband has "early onset Alzheimer's." In response, I
typically hear stories about dementia in someone's parent
or grandparent. For instance, a new acquaintance talked
about what it had been like when her mother was diagnosed with "Alzheimer's" (a term that is now used generally
for dementia or neurodegenerative diseases that may not

be Alzheimer's—a term originally used for dementia that occurs *before* 65 years of age) and had to go to live in a care center in her nineties. I hear about how hard it is to see and feel her mother's decline from being a well-spoken college English professor to being unable to recall what she wanted to say or had eaten for breakfast. Although I can see this is heartbreaking, and I know this person is trying to empathize with me, I am taken aback by the lack of congruence between her story and my experience.

Planning your future and sleeping nightly with your best friend and lover who is gradually becoming childish and irresponsible, as I said earlier, is fundamentally different from caring for an aging parent or spending time with someone who is old, frail, and demented. Caring for anyone who is ill requires endless patience, compassion, and sacrifice, but conditions vary substantially from situation to situation.

During the time I was first in contact with Deon by e-mail, Ed and I went through some intensely rough waters. One brutal day, for instance, a letter delivered by FedEx announced that Ed had lost his long-term care insurance. We were in terrible financial straits by then. I had just begun to make claims on his insurance for respite care for him. The insurance company claimed Ed had "lied" on the application he'd filled out in 2005 in which he stated that he did not have "problems with my memory." Ed didn't lie. He didn't know he had problems with his memory even though he worried every day about such problems. Early onset dementia erodes your trust in yourself because you are unable to see or grasp or understand what is happening. You can't hold the big picture in mind and you are unable to compare yourself accurately to a standard or a norm. This kind of dementia also erodes your spouse's trust in you because you use bad judgment, act badly, and cover all this up the best you can. Unlike most other illnesses—until the full diagnosis is clarified—there is no empathy or sympathy or understanding for what is changing in Alzheimer's, why it is changing, or *if* it really is changing. This fog of confusion fell over both Ed and me. For instance, when I first discovered what a mess Ed had made of our finances, I could not tell if Ed was exercising poor judgment and lying about the mess he'd made or if he was losing his mind. Neither of us wanted to reach the latter conclusion.

As a result of Ed's legal and financial problems, I had to hire a team of lawyers and Deon helped with this, both financially and emotionally. And so, I am grateful to Deon in countless ways, but especially for getting me to wonder why the simple exchange (without physical contact) of mutual witnessing is so compelling. All of us long to be desired, needed, maybe even used. We want to be provided for and supported and helped and cared about, but these longings are easier to understand. They are connected to tangible rewards. Your attachment bond with your child, for instance, guarantees you will try to keep your child safe, but it doesn't guarantee you will come to know your child as an individual. My friends' non-witnessing shows that even long friendship does not guarantee being seen. You might imagine that a parent-child relationship, a friendship, an intimate love and spiritual love are all different kinds of love, but I have come to believe they are the same love if they are the kind of love in which we can see our selves in someone else's eyes.

As I have come to discern it, true love is "one love": a space we enter with our beloved in which we reveal ourselves step-by-step with sensitivity, ambiguity, uncertainty, curiosity, noninterference, and without too many constraining assumptions. Within this space we come to know our selves and a specific other in a way that is fascinating and mysterious, a way analogous to how we come to know the tactile world around us, especially those aspects of it that are hard to discern at first glance.

Even now, I enjoy loving Ed and still take delight in him. On his 64th birthday, I ask him, "How old are you?" as I have done over the past 5 years. The question stumps him because he has no way to access any facts like that. I encourage him to "just guess" and he says with a very serious tone, "Between six and eight, I think." When I say he is 64, he laughs long and hard (and so do I) because it just seems absurd. I love Ed, but not as my partner. And I don't dwell in fear or sadness or anger (expressed or unexpressed) about this. I see how such feelings can create a narrative of self-pity or panic. Instead, I allow the feelings to be simply felt and then pass away. I encourage the story of self-pity to fall away. The more I practice this matter-of-fact acceptance, the more I can let excess emotion and reactivity slide off me like the cold water I repeatedly slip into on summer nights at my favorite black pond. It takes courage to move through that cold water in the darkness, but the courage increases my confidence and allows me to wake up to the present moment.

Ed's disease and its effects on my life brought a surprising desire to fall in love again. Over the decades with my husband, I speculated that I would never again seek an intimate relationship were he to die. I thought, "Well, I have had this one extraordinary love and I will never want another." Of course, in those imaginings, I saw myself as an ancient widow sitting in my porch rocker, listening to old Bob Dylan songs. Instead, I am still relatively young and vital. I notice every day how much I want a close and knowing witness, a curator of my own personal museum. I want to offer that to someone else, too. I am lucky to have had even one such person (many people never do), but now he is gone. Though I have learned to embrace solitude again (as I had in my childhood), I still long for someone to hold me and hold me in mind, someone to talk me into being, and someone with whom to stand on common ground and discover new horizons.

3.

I have always burned to see my beloved clearly, perhaps because of my being idealized and then devalued by my mother or because of my acute sensitivity to color and tone. The desire to know exactly and precisely what I love— people, places, ideas, and things—has been a drive all my life. The particularity of a person or a moment melts my heart. When I love an idea, I read and think about it constantly and I feel compelled to talk or write about it. When I love a movie, I see it at least three times (I have seen *Wings of Desire* at least 15 times). When I love a book or a poem, I read it repeatedly. When I love a song or a piece of music, I listen to it hundreds of times. When I love a person, I want to know him or her in all kinds of contexts and circumstances. I often wonder why other people don't repeat their most cherished experiences. Nothing is ever repeated

exactly because conditions (our perceptions, moods, surroundings, feelings) change. To see into the essence of what
you love, it seems to me, you need to know it under a variety
of conditions. When you can see into it and through it, you
see the whole world. I have come to call this practice "true
love"—the meeting of truth and love.

When true love involves two people, it provides a means
by which they can see themselves through each other's eyes:
a human mirror that reflects you in ways you cannot see or
know yourself. This mirror is based on trust—that the
other person wants to see you for yourself and will never use
that knowledge against you—that is alive, squirmy, indeter-
minate, subtle, and brave.

The scholar Stephanie Coontz, in her book on the his-
tory of marriage, shows how the relatively recent innovation
of an intimacy-based marriage has undermined the business
of marriage. Originally, and still in some places, marriage
was a social institution to serve the wealth and stability of
families who were, in effect, business corporations. Until the
late 18th century, most societies around the world regarded
marriage as too vital a political and economic institution to
be left to the free choice of the individuals involved. Marriages were arranged, often at birth, so that families, wealth,
and properties could survive; people thrown together in the
vow "Until death do us part" were mostly strangers or companions of convenience.

A huge unsung revolution has taken place as a result
of marriage becoming a personal relationship. Marriage is
now a relationship in which you can come to love another

person as a particular individual, and then your self as well. The features that make marriage an opportunity for development and self-knowledge also make it fragile and demanding because we are just babies figuring out how to love in this way. In my many years of Buddhist practice, I have noticed the absence of instructions or guidance in personal love. Buddhism guides us to feel and experience universal love—a kind of radiant expansive feeling for all things, an "aimless love," as poet Billy Collins calls it. Personal love—depending as it does on your knowledge and trust of your beloved—is in some ways more demanding than universal love. Many times I have felt a vast transcendent love that pops open my heart when I am on a silent retreat with a group of people who are personally unknown to me. But back at home, I can still become quickly frustrated when my beloved responds to me with the same repetitive or annoying emotional demands that are familiar in our relationship. Buddhist practices of mindfulness and loving-kindness may lack some spiritual fabric that would clarify a path of greater ease in personal love. Traditional Asian family structure encouraged family honor and loyalty, not personal love.

Knowing Ed in these recent years is a constant teaching about personal love. Before Ed got used to wearing adult diapers (which he's had to wear for about a year now), I would take him into the bathroom and say, "Now you need to use the toilet." Sometimes he would ask, "Which one is the toilet?"—being uncertain about the nature of "sink" and "toilet." Ed's inability to control his bowels and bladder was powerfully confusing and embarrassing for him when it began to happen as if out of nowhere.

I was in the bathroom with him just after he began wearing diapers and he was trying to urinate in the toilet. Standing at the toilet he says in a surprisingly clear way, "This is very hard." "You mean wearing diapers?" He nods "Yes." I say, "It's the Alzheimer's disease; it's not your fault. No one blames you," and he seems relieved. He finishes peeing and looks directly at me and says, "I never knew it would be this way. I am learning a lot." I sense the profundity of his remark. Years ago, I heard a story about a middle-aged man who was dying and clearly saw (in his mind's eye) some white-coated "officials" arriving to take down his Life Review on a clipboard. The man remarks quietly to his wife, "No one told me it would be this way." I know that Ed is saying the same kind of thing. In some palpable and simple way, he is a witness to his age regression and its mysterious effects on his being.

For me to love Ed in these past 8 years has meant that I am less and less concerned about "my needs" and more and more challenged to let go of him as my partner, my lover, and my friend. In order to love Ed now, I must become his mother, his protector, his advocate, and his highly idealized "good guy." He greets me now sometimes saying, "What a beautiful guy!" because he can't recall my name. I have sought out my needs for reciprocal love with others. Even a note of "sainthood" or false self-sacrifice on my part is an obstacle in coming to know Ed and me as we really are. To give to Ed *without resentment* is what I always aim to do.

The micro-aggressions still throw me: "I could never put my husband into care; I would care for him at home." "How can you deprive Ed of ever seeing again the rock walls he built in your backyard?" "Isn't it wonderful the way Ed adores you! He has always cared for you in just this way." When people say apparently well-meaning but deeply ignorant things, I simply feel my feelings—rage, despair, embarrassment, anger, hurt—and then let them drop away and work within myself to drop the narrative that would make these feelings into a story of anger, guilt, or revenge. Sometimes I say to myself, "People don't know my experience nor have they ever been close to a partner with early onset Alzheimer's." And, "I need to remember to write about this to let others know how much these remarks can hurt a caregiver who is trying to love and still be alive."

April 23, 2008

I wonder in a serious way about my own tendency to confuse needing me with loving me—all of my life. It started with my mother and has been an abiding confusion in my major relationships. In this way, though, I have developed a skill in listening closely and accurately to what people want and believe—something I deeply enjoy doing.

Now my husband is losing his mind. I am no longer in a conventional marriage, but I am devoted to his welfare. I am in a very complicated and multilayered setup here: Ed is neither competent nor is he old and frail. He is likely to live a long time, but in a very different state of mind than the ones he has inhabited over the years I have known him.

And so, I am in a bardo, a limbo, a transitional place in which I am trying to move through the confusion of what's before me as delicately and reflectively as I can.

I can imagine that Ed will eventually forget who I am, or at least put me into the category of "nice woman who is good to me," and already there's a bit of that as he totally idealizes me as a tremendously kind and good person and a totally attractive woman—without this being at all personal. It's hard to convey what it's like: He adores me and ignores me. I would not be able to live like this for a long time because his mind confuses mine. So, I am in a strange emotional landscape, unknown in many ways. I intend to be his caregiver until the end of his days, but I also want a life of my own.

The discernment I need now to love Ed, just as he is, means I keep my own counsel from moment to moment and day to day. When Ed first moved to care in early 2009, I sat alone in the dark for hours at night on many occasions, just to get to know the dark. I do this at the end of a long day of doing psychotherapy and/or visiting Ed. Prior to my living alone (on almost 600 uninhabited acres where there is no ambient light visible at night and no neighbor in sight), I thought perhaps I would be afraid and lonely if I lived here by myself. I thought I would be especially afraid of the dark. When the time comes, I decide to go directly into the dark and see what it's like. The dark is comforting and not at all overwhelming as long as I do not entertain foolish thoughts about "what could happen if . . ." I come to see there is a light in the darkness, a kind of golden light that is tremendously comforting and warm. I develop a friendship with the dark (and the light within it) and mostly I don't feel afraid or alone.

On one occasion, though, I am terrified. My lights and electricity suddenly go out on a summer night. I am talking with a friend in another state on the phone when it happens. He says I should call 911. I suddenly feel really alone, out here on the mountainside by myself. I grope my way over to the kitchen where the telephone base station is and dial 911. I reach the sheriff's office, 30 miles away. The sheriff stays on the line with me (because I demand it) and phones my neighbor up the hill. He discovers that the power company is at a nearby generator box to fix an electrical connection that had been damaged earlier in the evening by lightning. The workers turned off my power without warning me. Now they are walking around with flashlights in my drive-way. To be clear, I lived not entirely alone, but with a very large dog. Romeo had been mostly Ed's dog. At 135 pounds, this white American bulldog looked as though he could eas-ily take down a coyote or a mountain lion, but in fact, he was anxious and timid. As I talk to the sheriff, Romeo stands behind me barking. Even though he is a wimp, Romeo's size and companionship are comforting. (As I write this, Romeo is gone. He died in September 2012.)

Waking in early morning, recording my dreams, medi-tating and sitting at night in the dark (also swimming in the dark pond on hot summer nights) help me become my own brave companion. I find confidence and guidance in my own mind and through e-mail contact with Deon. Every day I ask myself the question, "What is life requiring?" I also steady myself by repeating, "There is only this and this and this. Now and now and now. Don't worry, dear (self). We will be okay." I allow any kind of self-pity to fall away. In those moments in which I might feel ashamed of having needs of my own or of not having made better financial plans, I simply feel the feelings and do not make a story out of them.

I rarely ask others what to do about my dilemmas because I notice that too often (1) they make up things based on little or no knowledge; (2) they give advice without offering to help; or (3) they engage in some kind of microaggression that upsets me. Instead, I decide to consult only those sources that seem to know something about true love. I begin to collect memoirs and poetry about love and to sort through them in terms of how good they are in discerning true love: a love that is always interested in the beloved; that is willing to be ruthless in perceiving the truth; that tries to "see" the beloved as a separate person in his/her own world; that knows reciprocity, mutuality, trust, and integrity are the grounds of loving well; that recognizes the vulnerability and risk we experience in being exposed to another's love; that, as a practice, attempts to tolerate and accept the faults and weaknesses of the beloved; that doesn't get steeped in rage or self-pity without a sense of humor; and that remains continuously aware of the profound mystery presented by the challenge to love and be loved in a personal way.

To investigate the ambiguities that still obscure my

views, I decide to make a "love pilgrimage": to visit those wise people whose work I am studying and whose lives have been challenged by love. Because my life has moved beyond *any* conventional scripts and love stories, I look outside of my usual places, even my usual Buddhist places (retreats, teachers, books) that I have come to trust. Most Buddhist teachings conflate love with compassion or with loving-kindness (friendliness), but, as I mentioned earlier, I have come to see that compassion and loving-kindness are not the same as personal love. Compassion is our capacity to suffer with another or oneself and to help in a precise way with that suffering. Loving-kindness is a kind and considerate attitude toward oneself and others. Buddhist teachings usually omit the importance of knowing the particulars of an individual—that experience of really knowing someone precisely, in glorious detail—as a part of loving them. And they also omit the importance of feeling mirrored and known by your beloved so that you can look into his or her eyes and see your self, make contact with your self. And the teachings don't help us see the ways in which our subjectivities become unconsciously entangled with our beloved, due to either an idealized or pathological symbiosis, an emotional habit, that usually comes from our earliest relationships.

And yet, Buddhist spiritual practices strengthen our capacities to concentrate and to accept our experience, just as it is. Two capacities are absolutely essential for building the trust and knowledge of true love: concentration and noninterference. If we cannot concentrate our attention and remain alert, we cannot remain interested in our beloved, observing the particulars. In order to see those particulars as they are (instead of as we want them to be), we also need the relaxed quality of equanimity or noninterference. A relaxed noninterference is at the heart of loving another in that it allows us to accept our beloved without trying to change or control him or her.

When Ed was evaluated with neuropsychological tests in the fall of 2007, I insisted we consult a specialist outside Vermont so that Ed's assessments could be kept private. As an indication of how much denial I had going on back then, I still thought there could be a possibility that Ed's disturbances were simply "neurotic." Ed was also hoping for that. We got him evaluated out of state and privately (even though it was an expense we could not afford) because we didn't want a neuropsychological evaluation on his medical record if he wasn't truly impaired. (The results showed that he had a serious cognitive impairment, having lost more than 50 points of his IQ and most of his executive functioning.) During the 2 days while Ed was completing 10 hours of psychological tests, I visited with my dear friend Joy at whose house we stayed. She asked about my life—something other friends rarely did in that early period. After Joy heard me out, she gave me a memoir by writer Abigail Thomas called *A Three Dog Life*. "Read this now," Joy said. "It will help you." I read it that night and it really did.

It's about Thomas's experience of her husband's dementia and death from a traumatic brain injury. The writing is alive, charming, funny. The book is about life and love, not loss. The book gave me courage and confidence that I would be okay even if Ed was losing his mind. I read it three times. I bought extra copies and gave them to friends. This book became my bible in trying to communicate my experience to close others. When friends asked how I was doing, I would ask them to read Thomas's book. Some friends actually did read it and got back to me to tell me how important it had been to them. I felt deeply relieved that it had been written. I could tell Abigail Thomas was a wise one. I desperately wanted to talk to her. In the summer of 2011, I got my first glimpse of her as I was driving in a light rain up her lane in Woodstock, New York. She was walking to meet me at a local café where we were to have breakfast and a conversation about love. In the way her body moved, I could instantly see the spirit of the person who'd written *A Three Dog Life*.

Abby's wide smile and her warm, friendly manner are completely endearing and we spent a lovely time visiting at the café and then in her dining room. When I ask her what she thinks permits us to remain interested in our beloved, no matter what happens, she says, "Well, I think there are some people that we are just supposed to be with. When we see them for the first time, we say, 'Oh, THERE you are! I am supposed to know you!'" Of course, I had felt this way about Ed when I first saw him in 1969. I feel this way about Abby as we are sitting together, but I can also see that Abby's life is overflowing and probably does not have room for a new friendship—at least at this moment.

Abby tells me about a friend of hers, a man whom she's known over many decades. She had felt this sense of karmic connection on meeting him. She's never had a romantic relationship with him and their friendship has survived a temporary break in her trust of him. When she eventually returned to him after a period of no contact, she told him, "I am not saying I forgive you because I don't believe in forgiveness." And he remarked, "You don't believe in it because it's the ultimate act of passive-aggression." Abby laughs hard at how well he knows her. It's his insight into her unconventional perception of forgiveness that lets her know that he knows her as an individual. She can see herself in his eyes. They resume their friendship. Abby remarks to me, "I think you can only forgive yourself, not someone else."

I find myself thinking about the fact that I never "forgave" Ed for all the trouble he's caused me: all of the financial problems over many years, and his earlier disorganization and poor planning that I had given up trying to influence well before we moved to Vermont in 1994. Abby remarks, "A friend sees you through all this calamity. He or she knows you in the familiar and in the mysterious. Calamity is the other side of the mysterious." Yes, calamity is the other side of the mysterious because it tests your love for your friend and your capacity to endure through thick and thin. If you grit your teeth and grind yourself down, you will not endure. If you can continue to witness your friend with the openness of noninterference, you will continue, but that requires love for your self as well as your friend.

When I gather with my closest women friends, we often remark that we can feel close and trusting even if we haven't seen one another for a long time. And yet, I have had breaks in trust with my closest friends, just as Abby had with hers. I can resume the friendship, though, when I see a friend's need and vulnerability and when the feeling of blame or control has been lifted. Old friends have a lifetime of knowing one another in ways that our parents, children, and even spouses may not know us. Ed and I were friends in just this way: Friendship seems to be the centerpiece of true love. Longtime friendship is, by definition, reciprocal, mutual, and egalitarian. It depends on ruthless honesty and relentless humor, and it is grounded in trust and integrity.

> *August 15, 2008*
> *Today I had a conversation with Ed about our sex life. Sitting across from him at the lunch table, I said, "I must stop having sex with you because of the changes that have taken place between us." Our recent lovemaking had had childish aspects in it that had caused me to draw back and recognize that I could not continue to have sex with Ed. I could not find myself in his eyes when we were making love. It was heart-wrenching to think about this withdrawal and gut-wrenching to speak about it, but I had to speak directly to Ed. I wanted him to know how much I loved him even though I needed to withdraw sexually.*
>
> *Ed looked crestfallen. "Are you angry with me?" he asked immediately. I replied, "No, not at all. I love you very very much. But there is a gap between us that is too wide for us to close." Ed responded, "Is it due to my cognitive problems?" I said, "Yes." "What?" I drew in my breath sharply and said, "You have lost a lot of your intelligence. I*

> *have not lost mine. There is no way to build a bridge across*
> *this gap. We have had a wonderful sex life and I don't want*
> *to spoil it." Ed looked solemn and reflective and finally said,*
> *"I understand. Thank you for telling me." Sadness and*
> *warmth pervaded the space between us as we held hands*
> *and cried quietly.*

Encountering the demands of loving Ed with less and less illusion, I think about the idea of a "gap" between two people who love each other. The gap is too large between Ed and me now. It is an impossible chasm. There is no way to build a bridge across it. Too small a gap often exists between people who cannot love each other: People are blind to the other's individuality, truth, and momentary being because they feel they *already know.* They are not mysterious or interesting to each other. Perhaps one or both people believe they don't need to ask what is going on with the other person. Oddly enough, married couples may idealize a state of being in which they "can just know" what is going on with the other person without asking, without taking the trouble to inquire into the actual existence of the other. In such a case—as is necessary between a young dependent child and a parent—communications are entirely by implication and intuition. This creates a problem of being emotionally entangled or enmeshed when it occurs between adults. You cannot know what is going on with another adult without checking. The notion of avoiding conflicts (by somehow feeling into the other person) is an impossible ideal. Having and feeling our conflicts (with respect) is a necessity, and there will always be conflicts. We have to see the particularity of the hurt and fear on both sides of the relationship. In this way, we create a "mindful gap"—a respected space between us. This kind of interpersonal space undergirds trust because we feel that we can talk to our beloved about anything without consequences that will be destructive to our love. Without such a gap, the other person often feels both emotionally managed and unknown as an individual. Never creating a mindful gap, and never valuing the other person's particularity, can keep some parents and children from loving each other over decades or even a lifetime, well after the child is an adult and the parent's equal.

Either the parent or the child (or both) remains caught in an illusion of overestimating or underestimating the other person. In place of love, there is control, obligation, desire for approval, despair about ever being known, or the deadness of uninteresting duty and obligation. Spouses can become mired in the same kinds of pathological symbiosis: They are bored when they are together, they set or keep ideals for each other (you should lose weight, stop smoking, meditate more), or they batter each other with unconscious emotional themes rooted in their childhood relationships.

A mindful gap between two people is an interpersonal space that is neither a chasm nor a merger. It's a mental space in which the other person can be truly witnessed—seen and known. In order to feel truly loved, we have to feel known as a particular person and then accepted without excessive criticism or correction. But this gap is absent when we fall in love, when we fall into an idealization (isn't she amazing, brilliant, perfect?) of the other person. Some people and some beings—like babies and puppies—evoke idealization. We fall for them easily.

Abby Thomas remarks, "As soon as you fall for someone—your baby, a friend, a potential partner—you are a sitting duck. It's like a virus. You need to recover from it as soon as you can because if you don't, it's just a pit. I realized that it's the same pit I felt growing up." She continues, "In order to endure terrors as part of life, you need to be your whole self—like it's okay to be just who I am and this is the best I can be. But that paralyzed feeling of 'I am NOTHING' comes back when you fall in love. You don't need it. It's like a vestigial tail. It's from the past and it should drop away." I like the way Abby puts this distinction between falling in love and loving another.

When we fall in love, sexual desire and physical attraction are usually driving forces. Fine. When you fall in love with your kid, you feel that narcissistic glow: "This kid is just like me, but better." Whether it's sexual desire or narcissistic fantasy, these opening forays into love are just that: a way to begin. The long journey of coming to know the other person as a unique and separate world—knowing that person through calamity and desire and conflict—takes place only after you can let those forays of your own desire drop away. Then you may be able to see your beloved without feeling an urge to give advice, make a suggestion, or pronounce a judgment. And that way of seeing your beloved will create a new desire to get to know him or her freshly.

Many parents idealize and mythologize their children so completely that they feel betrayed, as my mother did, when the child becomes someone who is different from the myth.

Loving Ed has, over the years, demanded that I perceive him as an entirely separate being whose personal habits (even before he got ill) typically irked me in the arenas of organization, ambition, and decision-making. In our first decade together, I tried to offer remedies and suggestions for "Ed's problems," but they never worked. Eventually, I saw and accepted that Ed was simply a much more disorganized person than I was. I came to welcome this less-than-perfect Ed. I enjoyed his company for his strengths and beauty: his warmth, charisma, charm, aesthetic intelligence, memory of poems and plays, humor, and spiritual yearning. I determined to allow the differences between us just to be and to work within myself on my feelings about these differences. Now that Ed has lost his cognitive and emotional maturity, I must do this in an even more radical way in order to love him.

To love another person in an honest and vital way, you have to be a whole self and permit your beloved to be a whole self, too. This is confusing because we tend to feel that we are "helping" our beloved by telling him or her how to change and why change is necessary. You know in your own bones that you are looking for your friend or parent or child to be interested in you as you are. You can read self-help books or go to therapy if you want to change; that is your personal prerogative, but it is not your parent's (once you are an adult) or partner's role. In Sue Graham

Mingus's wrenching memoir of loving the musical genius
Charles Mingus, *Tonight at Noon: A Love Story*, she struggles
to accept a man who threatens her and her way of life at
every level. In order to love Charles, she has to live separately from him. Charles is so overwhelming and "big" in
Sue Graham's life that she cannot inhabit a home with him
and have a whole self:

> I was hooked on his life, his music, his imagination, his
> passion and attention, his tall tales, his fury, his lies,
> his caresses, his extravagances, his lack of caution, his
> tenderness when he loved me and believed. I held on
> to that intensity without wrapping it up and sending
> it somewhere with a name and address. For years he
> would not forgive me for refusing to give our love an
> address. It was the source of every fight.

She loved him, but she couldn't live with him. Eventually, Sue and Charles did marry and move in together.

By not living with him in the early years, Sue protected
her love for Charles. What that means in my vocabulary is
that your beloved needs to be embraced—in terms of habits, desires, strengths, and weaknesses—and not subjected
to an internal review in which he or she has to be a certain way in order to underwrite your reality. If you cannot accept the other person as a whole being, then probably
that other person is not your beloved (even if the person is
your child). People are bound together in all sorts of ways
that are not love: attachment bonds, desire, passion, security

needs, power struggles, physical or financial or emotional dependence, or idealization. There's nothing inherently wrong with being connected in these other ways, but they won't produce the benefits of true love—of knowing and being known, of seeing yourself in someone's eyes and having your being enhanced through it.

After Ed received the results from the battery of neuropsychological tests, the ground between us shifted tectonically. I had to change my identity, too, in terms of what I needed and wanted and provided, in order to go on loving him.

> *April 24, 2008*
>
> *Tentatively and apprehensively, I want to have a new chapter in my life, one that is founded on a loss that I would never have wanted but also expresses the possibilities that my life might still hold. I must take things on where I have never been before, and I have some trepidation in going. I must look more deeply into the process of dying (for example, through studying Tibetan Buddhism) and see how my life needs to change in order for me to care for Ed and the others who depend on me while I go on developing toward death.*
>
> *Sometimes I feel tremendous anger and resentment about all that is demanded of me. I work within myself to let those feelings drop away. I almost never speak about them. With others, I feel protective of Ed and our relationship. When I am with Ed, I shower him with hugs and kisses. At the same time, I feel more maternal than spousal.*

Last night, sitting by the fire with Ed, he was reading and reciting favorite poems—Shakespeare and Longfellow—and it was just heart-wrenching. He cries so easily. He is so easily touched emotionally now by poetry. Oh my. I can hardly allow my feelings to make their way through me; they are so physical. My heart and my throat move in all directions and hurt me in indescribable ways. My meditation practice helps tremendously in allowing such physicality to penetrate me without harm. It's hard to find words to express the way these feelings move and affect me. I love Ed deeply and his childlike need for me is so appealing and so annoying. I am constantly hugging, kissing, and rocking him. What a time.

At the start of a romantic relationship we don't imagine a change as the result of which we would no longer trust our beloved to know and see us through no fault of his own. Ed's illness erased the key components of the love we shared: trust, integrity, witnessing, mutuality, equality, and reciprocity. Their disappearance clarified what we had. Love and control are opposites, it seems to me. It isn't simply that falling in love is out of our control—that it resides in the realm of karma, fate, or destiny—but that the activity of loving means the acceptance of your beloved without control. Often parents and children become badly entangled around the issue of control, especially mothers who need their children to be their friends or to be happy or successful. In my conversation with Abby Thomas, I say, "Hate and love reside so closely. My mother loved me so deeply and then hated me that much. I was alien to her for most of my adult life. 'Who is this person you have become?' she seemed to ask in horror almost every time we met. She never forgave me for becoming something so different from her. She wanted to have me as a close friend and she taught me how to be close and care about another's needs and feelings, but then she could not do that for me once I became an individual." Abby responds, "The hurt that repeats your first hurt hurts so much. My mother's focus was always my father when I was growing up." Abby's father was the renowned physician and science writer Lewis Thomas. "She would have been happier if she had had a job as a librarian or a historian. She went to Vassar for a year or so, and she was a passionate reader and absorber of culture. My father was very successful and a prominent writer, and I think she was very proud of him. When I was young, I wanted to be his muse, the muse of the poet. But when I got a little older, I thought, I'd rather be the poet!

"I got pregnant when I was eighteen years old and got married as a result . . . and I came to find out that I had married my mother because my husband would shun me for days on end when he was annoyed with me, just as my mother had done! When I was growing up, my mother made me feel guilty for the smallest slight or mistake. She'd stop relating to me sometimes for two weeks! During that time, I wouldn't even know what I'd done and so I felt it was I whom she was avoiding, not what I'd done. I think it's important, with the friends we choose and the parents we got, that we try to understand what they did, to accept it. If you don't do that, you become a bitter old crow. I look back at my mother now with the sense that we both failed. We were similar in many ways."

Developing a kind of "objectivity" about our beloved—maintaining a mindful gap between us—allows us to remain freshly inquisitive about the other person and about ourselves in the relationship. Sometimes we can't feel this about our parents until they have died. Only then are we separate enough to begin to get clarity about who they were. Ed's illness demanded a radical objectivity that I never imagined would be necessary in my love for him.

> *July 2, 2008*
>
> *I saw something about Ed this morning, perhaps more clearly than I have: He is unable to meet me, to share my experience, and he feels angry about that, as though I have abandoned him, whereas he has actually abandoned me. That's why our little pleasures (hiking and swimming) over the weekend didn't really help me. They don't cure anything. A nurse is coming next Monday to evaluate him for respite care. He is angry about it although he says he is willing to go through with it. Mostly I realize that I still hope for a sign that he is not losing his mind, that he is not becoming totally dependent on me. My life has lately seemed very stark, poignant, and something else . . . I don't know, maybe final. I have turned over every rock in terms of being "Ed's wife" and I am weary of it.*

Maintaining a mindful space between you and your beloved—not collapsing into an entangled merger or a chasm of being unknown to each other—requires the same kind of dedicated inquiry that a scientist uses to explore an object of study. Paying close attention and never losing interest, this is the way to develop true love. And it's the way we want to be encountered when we see ourselves in the eyes of our beloved: knowing and being known simultaneously—mysterious and newly arising. Coming to this discernment, I still have big questions about romance or romantic love—what a friend once called the "attraction of two limbic systems."

Romantic love has been idealized in Western cultures for what seems to be forever but certainly since our European Middle Ages. Doing therapy with couples for several decades now, I repeatedly notice how much people miss having a romantic story about their beginning, if they don't have one, and how much they draw a feeling of confident happiness from the story, if they have one. For example, if a couple says, "Well, we got together and got married because we got pregnant" and they don't feel the pregnancy was the product of some magical love, then they have an abiding doubt about the "validity" of their love even though they have been together for decades. But even the most perfect ideal of romance–"We met and locked eyes, and immediately knew we were soul mates"–is absolutely no guarantee of true love. Of course, Ed and I had that soul mates kind of start. All that falling in love does is set the stage for really getting to know the beloved; perhaps it makes us a tad more motivated at the beginning. I know now, though, that the important component of true love is not the romantic ideal, but the reality of staying interested in the beloved, keeping him in mind on a daily basis, in a way that guarantees he will be both familiar *and* mysterious, just like the natural world appears to us: familiar and mysterious.

What is the key to transforming the romantic event of falling in love into the practice of loving and being true to oneself and the other? I believe it is our skill and capacity to see and accept each other as separate, free, and different human beings. We must maintain a mindful gap between us—not a chasm and not a merger. From the friendly stance, "Plan your life as you see fit," we can always return to the question, "Do I see you clearly?" Of course, we don't ever do this perfectly well, but we can then talk together about the ways we struggle and fail because we trust both ourselves and the other person to engage in a conversation that is honest and kind.

If we cannot do this, or if we don't want to try it, then we need to consider the possibility that we are not practicing true love, but some other kind of bond with the other person. Sometimes clients in therapy ask me, "Do I have to tolerate his/her drinking, smoking, use of pornography, or indifference to sex?" First, I wonder why the question is put into terms that suggest a lack of freedom—Do I *have* to tolerate? When we think about how it is for the partner or grown-up child—how that person is trying to live and thrive or survive—we begin to look at the situation outside of our own feelings or longings or control. We also think about how it is for ourselves, tolerating these unwelcome habits or actions. Finally, we come to the point of seeing that accepting the other person, with a compassionate embrace, if possible, is at the core of loving. But if we can't do that now or ever again, the choice is always ours. Will you stay or will you separate, will you embrace or will you criticize, will you agree or will you disagree? We always have choices and that's why the bonds of real love are challenging, exciting, and, in their way, magical.

Most of us believe, though, that romantic love or falling in love is more magical than being in love. We like the flush of romance because it enhances our narcissism and makes us feel like the gods. Falling in love with a partner, a friend, spiritual teacher, or our own baby, we believe we have found someone who will complete us, be a perfect companion, or make us feel good forever. Of course, such a thing is impossible. Unless the other person is acting in a role that is not authentic or whole—being the perfect child, the perfect mother, the perfect object of desire, or the perfect provider—there is no "perfect" companion. What seems like magic when falling in love is the slippery aromatic oil of idealization, seeing the other person as "perfect for me."

When I studied the medieval folktale about the marriage of Sir Gawain and the Lady Ragnell (the story Ed and I used in teaching Dialogue Therapy)—in college and later when I used it in two of my books—I was intrigued by the premise it presents. Strangely for a story from the 12th or 13th century, it gives a very modern teaching: That we all want sovereignty: to be known and seen as having the right to our own decisions and lives. It uses the dilemma of the "ugly hag" being transformed into her beloved's object of desire (a beautiful serene woman). Will her beloved Sir Gawain choose for her whether she should be "beautiful by day in the court" or "beautiful by night in our chambers"? It is only Gawain's clarity—"This is your life and only you can choose."—that provides the great liberation and relief that tale has been building toward. The story puts this conflict about sovereignty and love into a nuanced context of magic spells, heroic challenges, and extraordinary insights about the nature of true love. When I go back to it, as I have repeatedly done throughout my life, I always find it hard to believe that it was popular so long ago. Why haven't we learned the lesson that the romantic ideal of a perfect other is not only false but also disrupts the spiritual and psychological growth that is naturally part of the path of love?

I decided to ask writer and teacher, Mark Matousek, his thoughts on love. I had read Mark's writing on the topic of love and friendship, and I knew he had struggled with love in his own life as well. Mark is a shiny-headed bald guy in his mid-fifties with an athletic physique, who describes himself as "bisexual." He is in a long-term intimate relationship with a man 7 years his junior. Mark begins our conversation by spontaneously distinguishing love from romance. I ask, "What is love?" Mark replies, "Fundamentally love is magnetism. It's the 'force that through the green fuse drives the flower.' It's the way we connect with each other and the world. How you use love is another thing, but love itself is the fundamental urge to connect." And yet, "the romantic myth destroys love because it is based on an ideal beloved. It is probably the most destructive story. Who can live up to its pressure? It's really only for the very young. The romantic myth makes no allowance for the waning of passion, of desire, of physical beauty. And it has tragedy at its heart in terms of always longing for the ideal. The more you objectify the other person, the less it is love and the more it is desire, passion, need, dependence. Desire may lead to love, but romance obscures it."

To love, Mark avers, means to look at yourself and your beloved in ways that clarify the reality of both. Spiritual teacher Cynthia Bourgeault says something similar in her book *Love Is Stronger Than Death:* "Love calls forth the reality of the beloved, and the act of loving calls forth one's own deepest reality." To love Ed over the years, I had to let go of all my strivings to be safe, heroic, or ideal. And now I must embrace the life story Alzheimer's has been writing, if I want to continue to love Ed.

In the spring and summer of 2012, I usually find Ed in his "girlfriend's" room where he spends the night and much of the day. It is touching to see the care given to him by this woman who is also demented and about 15 years older than him. She seems to have once been a beautiful and intelligent woman. Now she is a bit controlling and demanding; she wants to keep Ed to herself in her room. She doesn't want him to play with others. She dresses Ed in her clothes (pretty sweaters and colorful coats) and leaves him notes that he tucks into his wallet: "If you need me, just let me know. Don't let the staff ignore your feelings if you are sick." And the notes are signed, "I have always loved you." When I arrive to see Ed, he might be embracing her, but then he stands up and says, "Polly, darling!" They are both very happy to see me.

I am grateful that she sweetens Ed's world during the day and during the night. She adds vitality and new interest to his life. But then, suddenly, she must leave—move out of—the care center because she has been too dominant and jealous, keeping Ed from his activities and bossing the staff in regard to him. Her possessiveness creates problems for other residents, too. When she is gone, I miss her. Ed's functioning goes down a couple of notches immediately. Just after she moves out, I find him sitting on the floor in his room, looking like a small child who has been left by his mother.

True love, it seems, is a kind of "matrix" that underlies our emotional and spiritual reality. It has to be "obeyed" if we are to come to know our selves and our beloved. Love compels us to engage wholeheartedly with another person whom we need but do not control. This other person first magnetizes us and commands our desire. But then we must allow love to penetrate that desire and teach us how to remain openhearted with the stranger our beloved has become.

4.

In early May 2010, my 36-year-old son steers his old Volvo up my steep driveway followed by a car filled to the brim with stuff, only one headlight working, driven by his 77-year-old father, Richard. I already know the circumstances that are bringing them to my door. Richard, who has lived in St. Louis, has not been thriving for the past decade. Even though we have been divorced for 36 years, I keep close track of his life, partly because he visits my place on holidays and because we have an extended blended family in which my "wife-in-law" (never having been anyone's first wife, I needed a term that seemed friendlier than "your ex," so this is what I call Richard's wife before me), Richard's children (two of them are mine, as well), and their partners keep tabs on everyone. We are a friendly and somewhat nosey tribe.

Richard has been suffering from paranoia in recent years and this has been a concern of us all. His is an "encapsulated paranoia," and so he seems perfectly normal until the content of his fantasies are touched upon at which point he sounds completely crazy. Mostly the content has to do with Charles Darwin and the philosopher Daniel Dennett (really). The entire family has pledged never to use the word "evolution" when Richard is with us because it will launch him into a long-winded explanation of what is wrong with Dennett's theory of consciousness—a subject that Richard has written about and had some interesting perspectives on until it drove him crazy. Richard is by this time retired from his profession of teaching philosophy and works part-time for a real-estate assessor, looking at property and works of art to assess their value.

Throughout his adult life, Richard (who grew up in very difficult circumstances) has been plagued by something called obsessive-compulsive personality disorder, which means he is often obsessed about things in his work or his mind, he is hyperrational and overly idealistic and rigid in some parts of his life, and he is often irascible and increasingly paranoid now about subjects that might expose his vulnerabilities, including his lack of achievement. His personality issues also have led him to fill his house with items that should have been thrown away, and now his car is packed to the gills in the same manner. This "hoarding" is linked to his inability to decide what to keep and what to throw away, and so he keeps everything. Eventually the hoarding makes it hard to find what he is looking for and then he thinks someone might be stealing from him—Daniel Dennett and his band of rascals, perhaps.

Once our family did "an intervention" for Richard—a collective visit to demand he allow some of us to clean out his small houses (one in town and the other, an A-frame, in the country). By now the country house has been emptied and scoured and sold, but the other house is a fire hazard and Richard's mild cognitive impairment (early-stage dementia) means he is forgetful about leaving the stove on and the like. His very kind St. Louis lady friend, who was once his intimate partner, has been in touch with all of us about her concern that Richard needs care and can't any longer live by himself. While we are in the process of trying to figure out what to do, Richard takes the matter into his own hands and drives away from his dilapidated house with his "belongings" in the car (layered like an archaeological site with old file folders, photos, money, bills, some clothes, rotted food—you get the picture). He drives across country, sleeping a little in the car at rest stops, and shows up distressed, disheveled, and extremely anxious on the Massachusetts doorstep of my wife-in-law and her husband at a time my son happens to be having dinner with them.

We begin a collective powwow in which I want the role of "Medicaid expert" and "psychologist," but not "mother," in terms of what needs to be done. As it happens, the couple in Massachusetts (in their early seventies) feel they cannot make the arrangements for Richard's settling into a new life because the legal, emotional, physical, and social repercussions are too overwhelming. They hope Richard's children—in their thirties and forties now—can handle his situation. The "children" are all launching new chapters of their lives and no one can take Richard in and/ or do the research required to excavate his property, settle his finances (he hasn't paid his taxes for several years), and evaluate his mental health. Of course, since 2006, I have been dealing with dementia, Medicaid, care centers, and the National Association of Area Agencies on Aging (a very helpful organization).

I am still protesting when they arrive at my door: "Hey, I am overwhelmed with Ed's care and making a living. I can help, but Richard CANNOT stay here." Three hours later, I am staring Richard in the face and saying, "Okay. You can stay, but you have to follow my rules. You have to clean up in the kitchen after you eat and you CANNOT hoard or keep food in your bedroom." He agrees (of course). Inside 2 days, I can see that he is not capable of these simple tasks and that his cognitive impairment is bad enough that I should not pressure him to change his habits. His bedroom is soon layered with books, papers, food, clothes, and news-papers. He stays 5 weeks (part of that time, the other couple take him in also) and then we move him into a care center (about 20 minutes from Ed's care center; alas, I can't get him into the place where Ed lives).

So begins a new chapter of caring for another husband. Soon I come to have new respect for my young self, both in her decision to marry Richard and in her decision to leave him. I also find my way to loving Richard more than I ever did when we were married. Because I don't depend on him, I can see him now as a separate individual and appreciate his strengths—tremendous intelligence and endless wit, sensi-tivity to the sadness and constraints of life, respect for the underlying spiritual dimensions of impermanence and inter-dependence (he introduced me to Zen Buddhism when I was 22 years old), and a deep acceptance of moment-to-moment reality, including his own disabilities. I can also appreciate what life might have been like had I stayed with him: an impossible hoarding mess defended by abstract principles about his independence without any interest in my feelings or experiences.

Taking Richard in also makes me consider the virtues of "love on a one-way street"—or what I call "cherishing"—and to distinguish it from true love, which is mutual, reciprocal, and egalitarian (in case you've forgotten). "Cherishing" is the term I use for keeping and holding someone dear and cultivating your affection for that person. As I listen in psychotherapy to people talking about their children and pets and how much they "love and adore" them, I have come to distinguish such cherishing from what I have discerned as "true love," love on a two-way street. I see cherishing as different from mere "caregiving" in that cherishing has pleasure at its core. You definitely enjoy doing it or at least mostly you enjoy it. And that pleasure is definitely related to the fact that you come to know the other precisely and well. You come to know how to please and support that being. We can cherish our pets, children, parents, or siblings—without feeling known by them in a mutual way.

I totally enjoy caring for my new rescue dog (a spirited "red" cattle dog who weighs 45 pounds and is about 2 years old) even though she steals food from the kitchen counter and drinks half a bottle of massage oil. I contain my reactivity when she misbehaves. I don't beat her because she annoys me. Some people believe their dogs "love" them in return, but it is not the kind of love we expect from humans. Dogs are social parasites. They bond with us and get to know our habits because they need us for survival. Loving your dog is not love on a two-way street even though you may imagine it that way. Confusing cherishing with true love, as many do, keeps us from seeing clearly into both the real demands and the benefits of mutual love. This confusion damages our ability to love well and leaves us dismayed in life situations where we believe that cherishing another should be reciprocated, but it is not.

In the previous chapter, I mentioned the spiritual teacher and writer Cynthia Bourgeault and her memoir *Love Is Stronger Than Death*. Impressed by Cynthia's account of true love, I decide to seek out a conversation with her. Part of the year Cynthia (who is an Episcopal priest) lives as a Christian hermit in Maine and the other part of the year she teaches large public retreats. In the summer of 2011, I catch up with her at a retreat she is teaching at Wisdom House in Connecticut. Cynthia has an intense energy and concentration. She looks like a combination of an elf and a lumberjack, petite with an upturned nose and dressed in hiking clothes (having just come in from the woods). Immediately, I enjoy the clarity of her mind.

After about an hour in which we talk about the spiritual meaning of personal love, I ask her about parent-child love. "It is difficult to realize love in the parent-child relationship because of the physical and emotional needs of the child for

the parent and the parent for the child. Besides, parents usually prefer one child over another and every child feels this
and knows it. Someone is the parent's favorite. In my family, I was my father's favorite and my older brother was my
mother's favorite. No one knows what to do with this kind
of dynamic with a parent, but it is perfectly natural." Cynthia wonders if, by contrast, "grand-parenting can provide
a wonderful healing space in which the demands of parental possessiveness are lessened." The parent-child bond is
difficult because of the lack of mutuality and equality and
because of parents becoming enmeshed with their children
(and vice versa). "What passes for love with most parents
is the aggrandizement of the ego—a kind of narcissism
in identifying with your child." Meeting with parenting
groups and educators over these past 5 years to talk about
my book *The Self-Esteem Trap: Raising Confident and Compassionate Kids in an Age of Self-Importance*, I have observed
how hard it is for many parents to hold a mindful space in
which they see their children realistically or objectively.
Today's parents often idealize their children. That idealization may transform into devaluation after a kid becomes a
teenager, but in neither case does the parent get to know
that child as an individual. Parents may never know their
children as real people. It is also rare that adult children
develop a mutual love for their parents and get to know
them as people. Children have a powerful "archetypal"
(Jungian term for an emotional imprint) projection on
their parents and see them as bigger than life. Parents then
seem to be more powerful (even to a grown child) than they

actually are. To get to know a parent after you are an adult takes concentration, equanimity, effort, and persistence. The same qualities, of course, are necessary for a parent to come to love an adult child as an individual, neither dismissing the child's mistakes and weaknesses nor inflating the child's abilities and strengths.

Even to cherish a child, a parent must eventually come to see some of who the child is, in reality. Without that clarity about the nature of the child, the parent cannot see what the child really needs or how to provide it. There is a great deal of pleasure in cherishing another when we know that person in terms of actual strengths, weakness, needs, and character. We feel pride and joy in seeing our beloved thrive—in sharing in the other's happiness even if it differs from what we'd want.

Often I hear from my psychotherapy clients that they have had the experience of being totally unknown and unseen by a parent (perhaps even a parent who "sacrificed" for that child) who is wholly admired by the surrounding community. The grown-up child is shocked to hear from the larger community, perhaps at the parent's funeral, "what a loving person" this parent was and how much others believe "your father/mother just adored you." This situation is very confusing. This kind of parent-child "love" is not reciprocal; it is not felt and engaged on a two-way street by both people.

There is something deeply mysterious about mutual love because it brings us closer to the truth about ourselves as we try to see the truth about another. This kind of engagement is quite different from what I am calling

cherishment, even though cherishing brings us a lot of pleasure when the beloved is seen and known and embraced.
Still, it is love on a one-way street: We are not vulnerable,
openhearted, and in need of the other person's reflection,
interest, and desire.

When mutual personal love becomes a spiritual practice, remarks Cynthia, it means "baring one's heart with
particularity. This is the path of transformational love and
it puts a human face on the Transcendent." True love is
felt as a raw vulnerability with our own needs and desires
exposed. When it comes to being loved—not simply being
cherished or cherishing—we are touchy about how we
are seen and about not wanting to be used, managed, or
controlled. Most of us have radar for how we are seen and
whether we are being managed or used. Mutual love is one
of the few ways we can transcend our sense of alienation
and loneliness. Baring our hearts with particularity means
we will feel painfully wounded when our beloved distorts,
misunderstands, or ignores us. Wanting to correct the view,
we will make a bid for closeness by saying what is wrong.
When you attempt to tell your beloved, honestly, how hurt
and distressed you are about being misperceived or over-
looked—even if you have the skills of mindfulness—there
is usually confusion and distrust that have to be worked
through. Both of you feel uncomfortable and agitated. This
kind of interchange is a far cry from romantic fantasies
and ideals of an easy oneness or unity.

Cherishing—love on a one-way street—is a lot less
stressful and touchy than love on a two-way street. Some

of us learn early and well how to take care of the emotional and physical needs of a parent or older sibling on whom we depend. We can transport those caregiving skills into our adult relationships and enjoy cherishing others. But that does not mean we are open to true love. I have known people—even some "spiritually advanced" types—who have hidden all their lives from the exposure they would feel if they opened themselves to being loved. They are afraid of being known in this intimate way even if they long for it. My first husband, Richard, is one of those people; when we were married, he never openly expressed weakness, vulnerability, need, or gratitude.

In Richard's last chapter of life, at his care center, he has become a different person. He's been there since the summer of 2010. Since then, I have visited him about once a week with Ed. Early on, we would sometimes go swimming or shopping or for a long drive in the car on Saturdays. We always end our Saturdays at a small restaurant in Morrisville, Vermont, near Richard's care center: the Bee's Knees. And so, since 2010, on almost every Saturday night, you can find me at the Bee's Knees with Richard and Ed in a loose version of the "Mad Tea Party" from *Alice's Adventures in Wonderland*. There is little conversation and a lot of laughing, appreciation for the food, some sharing of Facebook material about our grandchildren and children, and a lot of nonsense that adds up to nothing at all.

In the early days, when Richard and Ed were more functional, there was pure warmth and pleasure between them: "Hey, bro," Richard would say. "It's great to see you!"

And Ed would give him a big bear hug. After all, they have known each other since January 1969. They have raised children together. They have shared a lot of winks, complaints, and warmth about their mutual friend (as the fortune cookie said), me. And now, they are sweet natured and totally accepting of their lives. These days, Ed is confused about who Richard is and whether we are saying hello or good-bye when we fetch him and drop him off. Still, occasionally Richard shows some impish competition with Ed, as when Ed asks innocently, "Whose jacket is this?" staring at his jacket hanging on the back of his chair and Richard responds, "Well, Ed, WHOSE would it be?"

Ed is not capable of playful competition, but he used to find it hilarious when I would announce, "We are going to pick up Richard!" When Ed was higher functioning he'd say, "That Richard is a funny guy!" By which Ed seemed to mean, "He is one crazy guy!" More than a decade ago, when Richard's paranoia was just shaping up, he and Ed were taking a car ride through the Vermont countryside, Ed driving and Richard riding. Ed said to Richard, "Do you ever think all these fears are just in your MIND?" and Richard quickly countered, "OF COURSE I have thought that! What do you think I am, CRAZY?!" Ed thought that this was just the funniest story because, naturally, he did think Richard was crazy.

Now we ride back together from the Bee's Knees listening on the radio to *A Prairie Home Companion*, which makes Ed laugh whether or not it's actually funny. We first drop off Richard at his care center. He says, "Good-bye, Ed! See you next week!" And Ed usually says, "Hi, Richard!" And we all laugh, and then I get out of the car and give Richard a hug and a kiss.

Richard looks me in the eye (at first it was shocking that he did this) and says, "I love you!" which he was loath to say when we were married. And then, "Thank you so much for all you do for me." It's a shock to hear Richard express gratitude and to feel his openness. What I did for Richard over the years was plenty, in terms of accommodating to almost no child support, always speaking well of him to our children, and providing a place where he could stay when he visited our children. His expressions of love and gratitude have now closed the circle around us and healed whatever was still sore between us.

Richard turned 80 in the summer of 2013 and that seemed to provoke a greater openness and need. He has fallen in love with a 73-year-old woman resident at his center, whom he's gotten to know through playing bingo and gin rummy (games he would *never* have stooped to in his earlier life). Last week at the Bee's Knees, Richard announced that he and she "would like to get married"! I about fell out of my chair. Richard has expressed a need for her company and a joy at having her as a close friend he sees every day. Strangely enough, Richard seems happier now than he has seemed in decades, maybe ever. He is warm and open and a little bit needy, and he gives hugs and says "Thank you!" If he had made these steps earlier in life, Richard might have been able to move from idealizing/devaluing his partners and children to actually loving them.

Saturdays with "the Dads" have become mythic. When

our children, friends, or extended family are visiting, they come along. We have interesting adventures—like when Ed had a vagal nerve attack and collapsed over the table at the Bee's Knees. Richard and I had to haul him up by his armpits and that was the first time I explained to the restaurant staff that these two guys suffer from dementia and that the younger one is really quite ill. Richard, Ed, and I ended up at the emergency room at the small local Copley Hospital. Ed's pulse and blood pressure were dangerously low. He had to stay overnight. I took Richard back and had to go fetch the dog, Romeo, from Ed's room and then return to the hospital. It was quite a scene.

Other poignant scenes, which have happened repeatedly at the Bee's Knees, involve Ed being approached by former patients. I see them coming up to the table and inside I say, "Oh, no!" Inevitably they come over and say, "Hi, Ed! Do you remember me? I am so-and-so and I saw you in therapy for three years" or "Oh, Ed! Hi! We are so-and-so and you saw us in couples therapy for five years. It was so helpful!" Can you imagine what it would be like if you approached your former therapist who stared at you blankly and said, even after you'd introduced yourself, "Do I know you?" I try to prevent such a thing from happening when I say, "Ed has Alzheimer's or Ed is cognitively impaired now." When Ed was healthier, he'd wheel around at me and say, "Why'd you say that?" and I would have to say, "This person needs to know." Ed's fans are always thrilled that he is still out and about.

The satisfaction I get from my cherishing Ed and Richard reminds me of the pleasure I get from doing psychotherapy: another example of love on a one-way street. I have been a psychotherapist since 1979 and a Jungian psychoanalyst since 1986. In the early 1990s, I quit my position as a faculty member of Bryn Mawr College and began to practice psychotherapy and psychoanalysis full-time. It may be hard for outsiders (those who have not participated in a long-term depth psychotherapy as a client or therapist) to imagine how much I cherish the people I come to know in my consulting room. It is an extraordinary privilege to be allowed such close access to the particularity of a stranger's heart. People do not come to psychotherapy to be loved, but to be helped with their suffering—trauma, addiction, adversity, and self-hatred, for instance—but I come to love them (not everyone, but many) because I know them so well and see them so clearly. I see them from the inside out and the outside in. The affection and concern I feel for them is similar to what I feel for my children: It is forever.

I noticed this fact years ago and decided then I needed to vet the people I would see in a long-term treatment. Once I knew I would often come to love them, I wanted to be sure I could also like them—meaning that they were generally truthful, at least a little bit openhearted, and able to give back to the world. This doesn't mean I am fussy about taking people into therapy. Jokingly, I might say I am trying to screen out the psychopaths and inveterate liars. What I really mean is that I will care about my therapy clients and cherish their individuality and subjectivity, and so I prefer if they are fundamentally trustworthy characters.

What does it mean that I am so affected by strangers

who come for help? Of course, we psychoanalysts like to talk about what is called "transference love" and "counter-transference love"—the ways in which we may be desired or desire our patients for neurotic or distorted reasons that are rooted in (their or our) unconscious fantasies of seduction, idealization, and power. Transference love certainly does occur in every long-term therapeutic relationship (and it needs to be interpreted and clarified), but so does real cherishment. Knowing the particularity of another's life story—the moods, habits, thought patterns, desires, and fears—makes that person lovable and compelling in the context of his or her existence. And that cherishment increases my pleasure in sitting with the person, even through the conflicts and rough encounters.

Wondering whether other psychoanalysts might share my view of therapeutic love, I talked to a couple of friends whose writings—especially about relationship—have been very meaningful to me. I wanted to find out if they also felt something uniquely precious about knowing their patients. I spoke with psychoanalyst and psychologist Nancy McWilliams by telephone. I have been in Nancy's company on several occasions: She is a slender attractive woman in late middle age. She maintains a full clinical practice and a demanding speaking schedule. I consider her a friend and I have great respect for her as a colleague. She is very well known in my profession because she is the author of several classic works that guide our field diagnostically and clinically. When I ask her, over the phone, about therapeutic love, she says, "Well, it doesn't feel qualitatively different

from other kinds of love, maybe it's quantitatively different. I feel maternal toward my patients. I am very curious
about their individuality and I am in it for the long haul.
Once I take someone into therapy, I feel this deep pleasure
in having found this wonderful unique person. It's a radical acceptance of the person and wanting that person to
be their very best self. It is very like parental love also in
tolerating the hate the patient might feel for me without
retaliating." Nancy's statement describes the kind of love
people everywhere desire: curious about one's individuality,
in it for the long haul, pleasure in one's uniqueness, radical
acceptance of one's experience and feelings, including hate;
and the desire for one to be one's very best self.

I wonder if the modern therapeutic relationship may
even have originated not from confession as Carl Jung
thought or from exorcism or mesmerism as several his-
torians have thought but from the development of the
intimacy-based marriage. After people were free to choose
a partner, they began to long for companionship—to be
seen and known as an individual. Some degree of leisure
time has to be available for people to open their hearts in
this way and the opportunities are always rare enough, but
such a relationship can be imagined and longed for once
the notion of it comes into our cultural consciousness. To
be witnessed as oneself, to be fully accepted and deeply
known, remains a more daunting task than contemporary
romantic or parental love can typically deliver, but perhaps
it is more readily fulfilled through therapeutic love with its
professional boundaries.

In another conversation about therapeutic love with a dear psychoanalyst friend, we looked briefly at a well-known early Western myth of transformational love: the story of the double-bodied creatures from Aristophanes, as detailed in the *Symposium*, one of Plato's dialogues. Deborah Luepnitz is a psychoanalyst and author whose book *Schopenhauer's Porcupines* is about the process of transformation in psychoanalysis and the challenge of therapeutic love. Deborah and I became close friends when Ed and I lived in Philadelphia, and she and I have continued our friendship over the years. We have talked about love on many occasions. Here is the way Deborah recounts the story from Aristophanes: "In the beginning of time, people didn't exist in single bodies as they do now. Instead, we were two-bodied beings, joined at the shoulders, tumbling around carefree, never lonely. Zeus took offense at these creatures who were self-contained and arrogant and showed no need of him. He rudely cut each pair in half to get them to show some humility. After that, each one stumbled around, vulnerable, miserably trying to find the other half of the self. And that's why we long for that one person—man or woman—who will complete us: Because in our true and original nature we were complete, not lacking." Deborah sees this as an allegory of romantic love in which we long for a soul mate. She adds, "The idea of being made whole by another person is an illusion."

Deborah, like Mark Matousek, believes that idealized romantic love sets us up for failure and self-blame. She also believes that romantic love is hyped-up because it is driven by economic factors: The more people invest in the romantic ideal of being the perfect object of desire and forever youthful, the more they will spend to make themselves attractive and desirable. Romantic love traps us in illusion and therapeutic love shows that it is possible to be seen, known, and understood without illusion. Therapeutic boundaries and ethical standards require that therapeutic love remains love on a one-way street. We cherish our clients about whose personal lives we know a great deal, but we don't reveal the particularities of our hearts to them.

Love, Deborah reminds me, requires a gap between two people. "One of my favorite contemporary stories (from Schopenhauer) about love is of porcupines who are freezing in the woods. They huddle up together for warmth and just as they are relaxing and feeling some body heat, they notice the pinch of the other's quills. They have to spread out again in order to take up enough space not to pinch each other. Then they get cold and they have to get closer again. This struggle never ends. If the quills represent aggression, there is no intimacy without aggression or hostility in it. The poet Molly Peacock says, 'Remember to make room in love for hate.' We have to make room in love for hate and every other emotion. We have to trust love to contain them all."

In fact, therapeutic love is designed to contain all sorts of negative emotions without retaliation. No wonder some of my patients declare, even at the end of therapy, "I wish I were married to you!" We therapists can resemble a perfect partner: We protect the space for deep inquiry. We accept peculiarities without blame. We never require patients to reflect on us as intensely as we reflect on them. When I was a young adult, I felt ashamed of grumbling about my mother's hate and envy or my father's delusions and prejudices. These things seemed trivial in comparison with the tremendous adversity, poverty, and trauma of my parents' childhoods—minor compared to the abuse that happened in other families I knew. But when I first entered analytic psychotherapy, I found my therapist was not only curious about my experience of my parents, but she also seemed to know it was possible that they were emotionally destructive even if they were "well-intentioned good people" and the "salt of the earth." It was a tremendous relief to be taken seriously by someone without having to explain too much or feel humiliated. I felt cherished by that analyst and have remained deeply grateful to her.

The therapist's cherishing of her patient, the parent's cherishing of her child, and my cherishing now of my dearest friend, Ed, and my first husband, Richard, are forms of endearment and affection that bring pleasure and fulfillment to both parties. But they are not the same thing as true love. They lack the mutuality and reciprocity, the experience of both people being on the line and needing each other in order to see themselves and the world. When we truly love another person, we cannot hide. We must open our own hearts as well as accurately witness another's.

The spiritual path of knowing and being known, of seeing and being seen was gradually made visible through Ed's Alzheimer's. Just as the spiritual path of celibacy or monasticism requires discipline, ruthlessness, commitment, and desire, the spiritual path of personal love brings similar requirements as you spend hours and days coming to know your selves in different conditions and contexts. True love opposes the control of your beloved while strengthening your need and dependence on the relationship for a foundation. This kind of spiritual practice demands concentration and equanimity, compassion and noninterference, but it does not end there. It means you see into another person so deeply that you can see through him or her to whatever you take to be the Divine Source, refracted back again through your own self.

In the words of Cynthia Bourgeault, "Our original desire to see and be seen is driven by Eros, a connective urge. This urge is the origin of the whole divine shooting match. It cannot be transformed by numbing it out. It can only be transformed by a bigger love—which means becoming a witness to another and yourself with your own open heart." In this way, she claims, we integrate individual subjective love (Eros) with transpersonal love (Agape). Only when the two are combined, according to Cynthia, can we truly know what it means to be conscious human beings: Consciousness is a relational field and personal love brings it fully alive. Many spiritual disciplines teach the separation of personal love and transpersonal love as though the former is inferior or smaller than the latter. My experience leads me to agree with Cynthia, who challenges this view. Personal love is a spiritual path that brings together the mystery of our connection to a specific other person with our connection to a transcendent source.

In these past 7 or 8 years, as I have been moving into my new life, some friends and colleagues have been surprised—

even shocked—to discover I wanted to live in an intimate relationship again. I have been confronted and questioned about my desire. Gradually I have come to answer in this way: Love on a two-way street is an ideal path for me for psychological and spiritual development. I have learned this from my direct experience in loving Ed, not from any principle or theory. Other peoples' experiences may have taught them something different: that celibacy, living alone, or living with a non-intimate friend is the ideal path for psychological and spiritual development. When I heard Cynthia talk about how she sees the integration of Eros and Agape, I felt excited and validated. "YES!" I thought. Now I sometimes imitate her language in talking about the spiritual challenges of personal love.

Loving Ed has required me to contain hate within love, unhappiness within tolerance, annoyance and irritation within humor, and difference within oneness. Loving Ed Epstein began mysteriously on an airplane in 1969 and continues today in 2014 as he regresses toward emotional and cognitive infancy. Loving him as an individual human being awakened in me a desire to clarify the spiritual matrix that commands us to know another precisely in order to know and accept our selves. Even when the matrix of love produces love on a one-way street, that cherishment breaks through the loneliness that dominates the human ego. When we are lucky enough to practice love on a two-way street, we truly come to feel that we belong here on earth and that someone else has been a witness to it.

5·

Although I was feeling alienated and unhappy with my second husband and confused about how to have an intimate relationship, had I not found Ed, I would have remained married. I had disrupted my children's lives with my divorce and I was coming to believe that being relationally deadened or embattled in marriage was the way "life was supposed to be." When I left my first husband, my mother was clearly ashamed and she stood right in my face and said, "Why are you getting divorced?" When I replied, "We don't have a good relationship," she countered, "A *relationship?* You're not in a relationship! You are in a marriage and you stay married. You take separate bedrooms if you have to!"

Of course, hers was the traditional view of marriage; it shouldn't depend on personal love. Those of us who grew up in America in the fifties and sixties were steeped in this view.

In my childhood, I saw my parents living awkwardly, resentfully, and sometimes disdainfully together. Usually there was a large chasm between them and a recognizable amount of zinging back and forth of small insults. When things heated up emotionally, the heat was conflict and pain, not intimacy or passion. Even as a young child, I could see they were not friends or even friendly with each other. In fact, if I had asked my mother if my father were her friend, I think she would have thought the question was ridiculous. Her friends were women. She felt comfortable with women and spoke openly with them about her complaints and hopes and dreams.

Until I was in junior high school, my mother did not drive a car. We lived in a rural suburban area on a dirt road. Her inability to get around on her own made my mother dependent on my father for more than income; she had to ask him to take her to the supermarket, her sister's house, and church. Many arguments ensued from these requests. When my mother told me, as she did on many occasions, "The only reason I stay with your father is for you," I wholly believed her and when I was older (in high school and later), I begged her to leave him because I felt she was miserable and oppressed. I did not think she liked him at all even though he sometimes reached out warmly to her to give her a hug or try to caress her. She always refused his advances.

When I visited my friends' homes, I didn't see any evidence of friendship between their parents either. Some parents seemed to fight less than mine did and typically their relationships involved less dependence on the wife's part: the wife drove a car and/or volunteered or worked a little outside the home. At my house, though, I could directly observe the suffering and agitation caused by one adult being dependent on another. As a child, I vowed independence, and my mother openly encouraged it on every level. It seemed that she said every day, "Don't depend on a man for your money. Get your education. Earn your own money." In those early years, my mother was my confidante and advisor. I took her plight and her instructions to heart. She wanted me to be her best friend as I got older and I was caught between my desire to satisfy her emotional needs and to have my own friends.

In my first two marriages, my friendships took place outside my marriage, just as my mother's had. I kept my personal views and desires under wraps when in conversation with my husbands. I studied my husbands and tried to understand them. I asked them lots of questions about their experiences, but I did not expect or get reciprocation or equal interest. When Ed and I became friends in the summer of 1982, we found we could talk about anything. There was reciprocation and equal interest.

Growing up in Akron, Ohio, I had had close girlfriends with whom I talked about anything that was on my mind. In my first 10 years with my mother, I talked about anything. My experience taught me that if I wanted a certain kind of meandering inquiry—moving freely through gossip, observation, humor, aesthetics, relational confusion, stupidity, intuition, and trivial longings—I should talk with a woman friend. Until I reunited with Ed, when women complained about men "being unable to communicate," I thought they wanted their boyfriends to be girlfriends.

But Ed and I had girlfriend intimacy; it included plenty of erotic desire and sex, but it did not depend on desire and sex. In other words, we could approach each other in anger or hurt or even resentment (feeling unfairly treated) and trust that we'd come around to feeling close and being able to solve the problems we were facing. We could gossip and tease and read poetry aloud and talk about deep philosophical issues (always my initiative) or the plot lines of movies or the troubles our kids were having or the blessings of family. Before Ed fell ill, we rarely said, "I want you to apologize" or anything like that because it was unnecessary. And yet, I don't want to exaggerate or inflate this aspect of our relationship. In conflicts, we were uncomfortable, snippy, entangled, and unpleasant to be around. Our relationship was *not* easygoing. And yet there was something ineffable and precious in its endless openness. We were always interested in each other. It was simply who we were together.

I know from my many years of Buddhist practice that the secret to a happy life is to remain interested in what arises on a moment-to-moment basis without too much judgment, anticipation, fear, or demand. If we loosen our grip, then life/the world joins the familiar with the mysterious and we are never bored or alienated. True love, it seems, must follow this path, *but* the obstacles to this kind of love for a particular person, on a two-way street, are impressive. Failures of love in marriage, parenting, friendships, and teacher-student relationships are legion and leave countless people feeling dead and alienated.

May 4, 2008

My relationship with Ed has brought so much trouble and anxiety for so long now that I look forward simply to greater clarity. My love for Ed is wholly destined. It has been strong and loyal and unswerving. Even though I have backed away from needing anything from him now, I still find him immensely dear, partly because I am losing him. Since about January, though, I have had a new determination to protect myself from disaster and being erased. Ed and I depended on each other for the past 26 years and now he is entirely dependent on me. I am going it alone and taking things step by step. Here we are about to face this awful shift in our lives and Ed comments to me, "This isn't so bad. I think things will just get better."

But then we were driving out to Craftsbury to look at the care center and it was a powerful emotional time. On the way, Ed was weeping and talking about how he felt he had wasted his life. He often says things like that now. We talked about our years together and then he didn't speak in the last 10 minutes of the drive.

The center is quiet, serene, and beautifully located—somewhat like a country inn. Ed immediately liked it and seemed to feel at home. We met a lot of people—including the cook who is a very likable middle-aged man who trained as a chef. Seeing the place seemed to give Ed some kind of boost.

When we were driving back to our house, we reflected more deeply on our years together. Ed said he regretted many of the ways he'd treated me—when he'd misperceived me, for example, alleging that I was "overly dependent"

on him. I asked him at one point what he thought had
happened. He replied, "Envy." He said, "You were always
too far ahead of me on the path. You outperformed me on
all kinds of tasks from the intellectual to the spiritual."
This is not really true, but it was the way he was seeing it.
He also said he grew up a level or two to be with me—to
a level he wouldn't have otherwise reached. He expressed
warm gratitude for what I have offered him and how I
have taken care of him. We cried a lot and the afternoon
was very tender.

In 2009 and 2010, I began to teach workshops about
love and desire, trying to discern what I began to regard as
a "sacred path from desire to love itself." For decades, I had
written and taught about "desire" as the restlessness that
comes from the feeling that something is missing; desire sep-
arates us from direct awareness of our immediate experience,
takes us off track from our concentration. But it also orients
us to what we want; it's just that we need to recognize we have
it when we get it. If you have no knowledge of what you want,
you won't know it when you get it. If you have never known,
for example, high-quality chocolate, you can't really recognize it when you get it. Desire arises when we have had something that satisfied us and now it is missing. (Of course you
can wish for things you've never had, but that wish is based
on fantasy until you've actually had the experience.) Now that
I had lived within the vitality and freedom of a loving relationship, I want that kind of relationship again although it
cannot be with Ed, and I don't know if that will work with
someone else.

Ed and I spoke plainly about our "karmic connection" and our "devotion" to our love. Over the years, Ed said many times that if he died first, he would want me to live in a relationship again. He said, "You'd need it; you are very relational." In my love pilgrimage, I am trying to discern the nature of love—a love that has spiritual and psychological components—and I am also hoping to find out if I can love again.

When I wrote *Women and Desire: Beyond Wanting to Be Wanted* in the late 1990s, I studied psychoanalytic and Buddhist teachings about desire. Many people have the impression that Buddhism condemns desire, but that is not true. Buddhist teachings ask us to stem or eradicate what is called (in English) "craving and grasping"—a blind drive or thirst that is exemplified in addictions, restlessness, and our desire to control our own and others' lives and circumstances. Many good parents, for instance, mistakenly grip on to their children's "happiness" and feel driven to "give them every possible opportunity for success." This creates the grasping kind of desire that can eventually alienate the children.

I see this kind of desire finally fading within me as a parent now that my life has changed with Ed's illness. When my mother said that Richard and I should take separate bedrooms so that I could stay in my marriage to him, she said it, no doubt, for my "own good." She thought this would make a better life for my children and make me happier as a result. She had decided to stay with my father for my sake, even though she didn't really love him. Imposing our ideals or our fantasies on others, no matter how important they seem, leads to misery. We lose our flexibility to know that other person just as he or she is.

On the other hand, our intentions and desires are very important for our lives. They allow us to give a meaningful direction to our actions and plans. Too many times, we all (especially women) try to appear in a certain desirable light—beautiful, nice, good, helpful, kind—and hope that someone *else* will see us that way and love us for it. Such attempts to become another's object of desire lead only to resentment and bitterness. You have no implicit contract with another in which that other person can become responsible for your happiness. You have to be responsible for your own happiness even though you don't control it.

Cherishing Ed through his decline has freed me from trying to put on appearances. My life does not fit into conventional roles and models. It's hard to say exactly whether or not I am "married" to Ed; I am divorced, but I am also devoted. But then, I have been divorced from Richard for almost 40 years and I cherish him and help him! The other day Richard said that his friend was "confused about why my former wife would take me out to dinner." I don't even know what "former wife" means any-more! Still, I want to be seen and known by others in a way that helps me know myself; I am not grasping at being seen in a particular way, but simply at wanting to be known by others. For the Christian hermit Cynthia Bourgeault, being witnessed—for who we are and are not—is the very crux of giving and receiving love as a spiritual practice. Cynthia says, "The division between personal and spiritual love is a fundamental mistake." If we can focus our awareness on baring the tenderness and sadness of our own hearts and receiving that of our beloved, we begin to move along the spiritual path of love.

Although love is in its essence personal, "the human passions are impersonal," Cynthia says. Our sex drives and attachment bonds and our drives for power are "passio"—they act on us and we act them out without discernment; we lose our discernment when we are swept up into our passions. When we are swept away, we lose track of our own particular being and we are also blinded to the reality of the other person. At these times, we tend to use the other person to meet our needs instead of experiencing them as a separate person interacting with us. Of course, in lovemaking and playing, we sometimes "use the other person" in a mutual and consensual way, but that is different from ignoring the subjectivity—the emotional being—of the other.

In addition to her study of spirituality and religions, Cynthia draws on a unique personal love relationship with a 72-year-old Christian monk, Brother Raphael. They met at a monastery and Raphael fell in love with her. "The desire to see and be seen was intense and voracious and possible" with him in a way it had not been in her two marriages. Many religious teachers and monks "hide in the impersonal" when it comes to love, says Cynthia. They try to develop a transcendent or universal love and cut themselves off from experiencing the erotic impulse to connect in a particular and personal way. True love—love on a two-way street—demands the involvement of both partners for this reciprocal witnessing. "Eros is personal and particular. It naturally transforms into Agape—universal love and openheartedness—by going through the fire of being vulnerable to another person," Cynthia says. "It can only happen if you allow someone to entrain your erotic desires in a way that does not involve simply acting out your passions." I think about the many ways in which Cynthia's ideas add something new to spiritual accounts of love. Too often in Buddhist contexts, for example, I see the emphasis on compassion, loving-kindness, and friendliness as a kind of universal practice without any attention to the "entraining of erotic desires" in a way that leads to embracing another individual as a particular person.

When I began my love pilgrimage in early 2010, I wanted to speak with the poet Naomi Shihab Nye because her poem "Kindness" had been medicine to Ed and me during the early days of Ed's illness. He and I had read it to each other countless times. Of course I know and love other poems by Naomi also, but "Kindness" convinced me she knew something about the love I was trying to discern.

Though I wasn't able to meet her in person, we had a warm conversation by phone. She spoke at first about an unusual reunion in her childhood St. Louis neighborhood with 10 other people with whom she had played in her youngest years. In this adult reunion, they shared the details of experiences that were too painful or humiliating to talk about when they were children. Naomi noticed "how much more intimate we felt because of the secrets we revealed."

Witnessing these previously hidden sufferings brought her friends back into one another's inner circle after many decades had passed.

Then Naomi shifted her lens to a bigger view of love. She said that part of the reason these strangers, these friends from long ago, were so important to her was that they connected to a time in her life when she felt acutely attuned to the beauty of the world. Like the poet William Wordsworth who recalled that in his early years "The earth, and every common sight," seemed "appareled in celestial light," Naomi saw the extraordinary in the ordinary.

> In my youngest years, in my early childhood at ages 3 and 4, I felt an overwhelming tenderness towards life. I knew it was utterly precious. I saw that it was an impossible miracle that there is anything here at all and that we are here to witness it . . . I remember this extreme state of wonderment. I just wanted everyone to slow down and be present to that wonderment. I remember thinking at age 3, "It is a miracle that we are here. See: this grass, these trees." I was overwhelmed with these feelings . . . I remember still the way the light would fall on the street, on our doorsteps. I remember these details still and I really think this was why I became a poet.

I asked her why she thought it is so hard for people to love others in their families and marriages over time with this same sense of wonder. What is the obstacle to experiencing the miracle of being together? "I don't know. It is very hard. The room of the mind is cluttered with doubts, remorse, frustration, disappointment, and desire. All of this takes over and blocks out the mystery." Ed and I felt we were "living inside a miracle" as though we had been selected for each other by a mind or an impersonal force that knew us before we knew each other.

Talking with Naomi and Cynthia, I remember how Ed and I loved to reminisce about our unique beginning and our amazing reunion. Somewhat sheepishly, I also recall how these conversations included our making fun of "the French" (our stereotype, no doubt) and their insistence that there was an inherent alienation and isolation in human life. Ed and I had separately been students in France during our college years and perhaps we were reacting to the whiff of superiority we had felt from many French people in those post–Vietnam War days. Still, from the time of philosopher René Descartes and his writings on doubting our subjective experience, the French had, we believed, been trying to think themselves into feeling that palpable sense of union. Maybe most people believe we are "strangers in a strange world" and that we can never really see or know one another. The insulation of our subjectivity—Do you see the same "red" that I see?—seems to be an immutable truth. Equanimity with those differences, however, and the desire to see and know another person in the same way you want to study the natural world—to come to know it in itself, not simply as it seems to you—can allow you to accompany another in need, vulnerability, suffering, and limitation, and also to reflect the particular strengths, beauty, and talents of that other.

Two days ago, I was sitting across the table from Ed, having pizza. Between taking big bites and saying "Mmm," Ed stared at me, his huge brown eyes looking very much like the eyes of a 2-year-old admiring his mom. Ed was very happy to see me. I was also happy to be seen by him in this simple way. About a month ago, we were having dinner with other family members—a table that had six others seated around it, including me. We were all chatting and Ed was just laughing, sometimes repeating words I said. Then at one point, my stepson's wife, Sarah, asked Ed a question. I don't recall what it was. Ed responded with a gibberish word salad that had intonations and pauses sounding as though he was answering her question. Then he stopped and said clearly, "I really don't know who I am!" I think he meant to say, "I really don't know what I'm saying," but what he actually said felt profound.

My fundamental connection to Ed leaves me speechless. And yet, I want to emphasize that the miracle of our love has never been easy or even always habitable. It's like standing in a cold waterfall that runs sometimes very heavily and sometimes lightly but is always shocking. Caring for Ed (and Richard) in the way I do has heightened my desire to see love as distinct from idealization or any kind of aggrandizement. Love requires a spacious perspective and it also demands reciprocity: that *both* people are in the relationship with the desire and intention of knowing both themselves and the other person. Otherwise, what we take to be love is cherishment at its best and propaganda at its worst.

Apropos of cherishment versus love, I met up in a

café in New York City with my friend and colleague Pilar Jennings, a psychoanalyst and Buddhist practitioner who teaches and writes about the power of relationship in Buddhist practice and psychotherapy. With her bright blue eyes and curly auburn hair, Pilar looks younger than her midlife age. She wanted to talk about how she has transformed her relationship with her parents as an adult. She began by speaking about the "oneness" aspect of love: that feeling or experience of being "one with your beloved." She commented, "In the parent-child relationship, parents have a natural tendency to meet their own narcissistic needs through their children, wanting the children to be happy and successful. But the desire to control the child creates a difficult situation. You need mindfulness to enter into another's subjectivity and to allow whatever is there. Everyone has the opportunity to love their parents, if they grow old together, but it was my spiritual practice that allowed me the spaciousness to do so. At an age when the obstacles were gone enough, I began to step back and see who is the person of my mother, my father. I really said, 'Who are you?'" I mention to Pilar that I am trying to distinguish mindfulness from love. Mindfulness is the skill of working with our own experience—being attentive, clear, and accepting—but if it were the same thing as love, then all those who are skillful in mindfulness would be skillful in love. That is hardly the case.

In order for a mature love to develop between two people (for example, a grown child and a parent), both partners have to be ready and interested to know each other, to know the particulars, and to hold each other in mind. The desire to know the other person as an individual distinguishes love from mindfulness. Sometimes the parent wants to get to know the child as a separate person and the child does not reciprocate in wanting to know the parent or even in wanting to be exposed to the parent. But if both people are ready, such a development is tremendously rich and beneficial for both, and for the family in which they are developing. This brings to mind something my psychoanalyst friend Deborah Luepnitz said to me when I talked with her about love: "In *The Philadelphia Story*, Katharine Hepburn says, 'The time to make your mind up about people is NEVER.' That's probably as Buddhist a statement as any about love."

To look more deeply into Buddhist "statements about love," I met with Shinzen Young, my Buddhist teacher since 1996. He knew Ed and me as a couple, beginning in 1996, and witnessed the changes between us as Ed got ill, moved away, and has continued to decline. In the summer of 2011, Shinzen and I converse at my home in Vermont where he is going to lead a daylong retreat on the following day. In the background, Hurricane Irene rips through the countryside. Shinzen has been married and divorced and his ex-wife just happens to be sitting in the chair next to me as he and I talk about love. She and he are still good friends.

Shinzen stresses the oneness or unity aspect of love, a universal spiritual perspective on love. He says, "Love is the experience of another as a non-other; you become the other. In that moment, you are having a complete sensory experience of the other—with no need to push or pull on that experience. You could say love is synonymous with equanimity. In such a state, there is no subjective reaction that the 'other' exists; it is entirely 'I am the other.' You are merging with the other and your center of identity is the other." This is not confusion between self and other, but a joining of the perceptions of "self" and "other." Not a desire to control or incorporate another person into your identity, this kind of oneness is simply your total openness to seeing/feeling/hearing the other person as she or he is. You drop the distinction of "you" and "me" and the defensiveness that goes along with it.

Shinzen continues, "After you have had this kind of experience with another person, then you have thoughts and feelings about the other person that are conventionally called 'love'—'you are so beautiful,' 'I can relate to you,' 'you are perfect!' But when you are having the experience, you are just having it. You don't exist as 'I' because there is a safety in not having to be a self; what is reflected back is not myself, but an impersonal state of absolute safety. Love, as we conventionally describe it, arises AFTER the experience of oneness or unity."

This transcendent love is a goal of spiritual development in many meditation traditions—a love that can be felt anywhere with anything. In this account, love is on a one-way street. It is not a reciprocal account of two subjectivities, but an account of only one.

Here is how Shinzen breaks down the phenomenon:

1. Perfect equanimity with other—complete acceptance

2. Experience of other without any subjective reaction—neutrality

3. When subjectivity arises, the other is me and I love it

4. Identity shifts to other

5. Other and self arise together flexibly

6. External world arises as pure "expansion" (outward movement and openings) and "contraction" (inward movement and closings)

Shinzen avers that the oneness or unity aspect of love is a kind of "zero" (vanishing) between expansion and contraction. (Some aspects of an orgasmic climax are like this vanishing in which time and space seem to collapse and form again.) Spiritually, we experience the non-separation from the beloved as evidence that we are not ever really separated from anything. This kind of love is at the heart of enlightenment; it gives rise to endless compassion for the world, our selves, and others.

On a practical level in a human relationship, when you commit yourself to the inevitable changes in a relationship with a particular person, you get indispensible feedback about your ability to rejuvenate your love. If you can return to this oneness, then you can follow your love as a spiritual path. Shinzen says, "If you can really know and accept your beloved, you will not suffer from the differences and upsets between you. And you will also find that the Divine Source comes right through your relationship—an engagement with divine love." Although Shinzen uses terms that are somewhat different from Cynthia's, I think they are talking about the same phenomenon. But Cynthia emphasizes that the process of Eros becoming Agape is on a two-way street; it is mutual and reciprocal.

Many of us imagine the unity or oneness aspect of love as easy and comfortable; we think of it as an easy fit between two people. Occasionally this is the case, but often the experience of unity paradoxically emerges from the differentiation of the two individuals. Sometimes it is the mindful gap between two people that allows them both to feel joined, accepted, and known. Inside the space of encountering your beloved, there may be strong feelings of anger, frustration, hatred, jealousy, or competition, but the connection allows these feelings to be transformed into warmth, gratitude, and love.

My friend Mark Matousek says it this way, "Love is actually intensified because there is a kind of paradox working on us: Because we recognize the imperfection and the impermanence of our beloved, our experience is more precious. It's like the cup that is already broken in your mind's eye while you are using it. You feel more connected because you know your love is already broken." I have often said that love is a spiritual training for a broken heart. Your heart will break if you love someone. Something will happen to one of you—illness, accident, separation, betrayal—that will result in loss and pain. But the truth, the witnessing, and the oneness can transcend that loss and transform it into a spiritual adventure—the spiritual adventure of being human. To be as clear as possible, though, I have found (in working with couples and individuals in psychotherapy) that betrayal creates emotional states that are harder to transcend than the states created by other types of loss that are not rooted in blame. Because betrayal breaks our trust in our beloved, we can get permanently caught up in fantasies of retribution and feelings of shame and humiliation. I have not been betrayed in my own love relationships, as far as I know, except in the way that my mother reversed her early love into later hatred. But her reversal was not a matter of lying to me or humiliating me. I could still see my mother compassionately and embrace her warmly with her faults. But I have learned about betrayal, in great detail, through working with others in clinical settings. I have become aware that betrayal exists in its own category of broken-heartedness because it may prevent you from embracing your beloved as a whole person or your self as a whole self. Because reciprocal trust is the underlying fabric of true love, when that trust is torn, it may feel impossible to restore it even though you can see your beloved's faults and other imperfections.

When you love a particular person, all of their faults, limitations, annoyances, and shortcomings are included in your affection. Over time, as you really come to know those faults and shortcomings, they become part of what keeps you fascinated. Because you want to be close to the other, you are motivated to develop acceptance and equanimity in the presence of faults. Mark says, "You have to get over your annoyance in order to really love. And your beloved is the best motivator for developing this kind of acceptance—the basis for spiritual practice—because he or she really irritates you. Giving up your desire to control or change the other person is a sacrifice you make for love. 'Sacrifice' has become a dirty word in our culture, but to me, love without sacrifice is not really love."

The impulse to love is in all of us. It expresses our intuition that there is an underlying unity in our experience and that we are never separated from the world in which we are embedded: Love is our true matrix. Our individual experience of this unity is our unique attraction to another person. That attraction gets us through the door of love and we have that initial sense, as Abby Thomas put it, of "Oh, THERE you are!" and it feels also like "Oh, HERE I am!" In order for the spiritual path to develop and deepen, we have to commit ourselves to knowing, accepting, and loving that particular individual with all his or her strengths and weaknesses, needs and, desires.

Mark continues, "When you commit yourself to loving just one person, you have to engage in what you love and what you don't love. You don't have a different person for every desire. I see this as a spiritual matter. Just as Meher Baba said, 'Dig in one place.' If you try to do ten spiritual practices, you won't do any practice. It's the same with love. To bore down into it, and overcome what life challenges you with, makes love more precious. And it always includes loss, pain, struggle, imperfection, and the ways the other person doesn't satisfy you and never will. This kind of love is messy and difficult and that's why a lot of people can't do it."

As you bore down into your love, it also has to be mutual: Both people need it and depend on it for their confidence in being in the world. This does not mean some glued-at-the-hip codependency. But it does mean vulnerability. You come to recognize how important your beloved is in helping you see your self and in giving you a different view of the world. You want to see your self more clearly through the eyes of your beloved—in addition to whatever you want to offer for helping and supporting the other person. In the process of mutual reciprocal witnessing, the help that each person needs, and the attention that each gives, emerges moment by moment and changes over time. In my relationship with Ed, the distribution of help and need was never fifty-fifty. When love is on a two-way street and it is moving along that avenue, the two people see their help and care and interest going back and forth, not fifty-fifty at any given time, but balancing out over the years and decades. Otherwise, the relationship will not be love, but cherishing or dependency or fulfilling of roles, as my relationship now is with Ed.

In order to know our selves, and our common humanity, we have to know another as a particular being. To love in this way, we must also feel our dependency on a valued other with his or her weaknesses and limitations. Cynthia's friend Brother Raphael had not allowed himself to be vulnerable in this way prior to meeting Cynthia when he was 72 years old. Until then, he was striving for a pure and perfect love—a love of God—and had not bent down to loving another person who could also see and know him. It was a risk he took finally at the end of his life.

Tragically, much spiritual abuse has unfurled under the banner of transpersonal or impersonal "spiritual love" in which an idealized spiritual teacher or a beloved priest or minister offers a distorted gesture of intimacy or physical closeness, taking advantage of his role. What is always missing in these cases is the vulnerability of the person in the powerful role. That person does not feel a reciprocal love in which he bares his heart with its particularity. Perhaps it is a good rule of thumb to keep in mind: The spiritual path of true love should feel mutual and egalitarian for *both* people, each exposing the tenderness of the heart. In the process of opening our selves to true love, we come to see what it means to become conscious of "self" and "other" and to accept the space between us. As we stay connected through our hurts, angers, and differences, a unity develops that allows us to live inside a miracle.

6.

In late December 2012, I am on my way to Bodh Gaya, India, to take a 10-day Tibetan Buddhist retreat on "conscious dying"—an ancient practice called *phowa*. Ed's illness has all along brought a new investment on my part to learn about dying. In the spirit of being fascinated with what is inescapable, I consider death to be one of life's greatest adventures. I want to encounter it wholeheartedly and to help others, especially those close to me, to do the same. The obstacles to dying well are many and sometimes insurmountable, but I have enjoyed learning all that I can about it. Accompanying my parents in their dying was—both times—a profoundly transformative experience. They both died well and peacefully in their mid-eighties; their deaths took place in the late 1990s. They still serve as an example to me of dying without regret.

Going to India to take this retreat on conscious dying is at least a step or two beyond my comfort zone. I have previously taken this same 10-day phowa "course," as it's called, with the great Tibetan Buddhist master Ayang Rinpoche, who is teaching it in Bodh Gaya. The first time was at the Garrison Institute on the Hudson River in upstate New York. That was 6 years ago: Ed was still living at home then. He was being watched over by friends, and I had no phone contact with him or my home while I was on retreat.

Back in December 2008, I plunged into the phowa retreat and turned a corner sharply in my life. Both within the retreat and after, I had a sense of becoming truly and deeply unknown to myself. The retreat exposed in my own subjective experience what the Tibetans call a "mindstream" underlying my surface identity. I lost a sense of myself being simply "Polly." At the end of his life, and at the end of his autobiographical memoir, *Memories, Dreams, Reflections,* Carl Jung says, "There is nothing I am quite sure about. I have no definite convictions—not about anything, really. I know only that I was born and exist, and it seems to me that I have been carried along. I exist on the foundation of something I do not know." At the 2008 phowa retreat, I had a palpable, even personal, experience of existing on a foundation of other lives, dedications, and efforts that were not mine. These were my spiritual ancestors, not my biological ancestors. I could feel how I had benefited from others who had contributed and accumulated sensitivity, knowledge, and insight in lives before this Polly life. I could feel distinctly how my life was not my own. This was new territory for me.

Phowa is a yoga-like energy practice in which one learns to bring one's consciousness up to the highest chakra (the top of one's head), as a means of practicing a method that can be used in the actual dying process. If one is skilled, one may be able to avoid the *bardos* that typically occur after death. These bardos are predictable transitional states between dying and rebirth (or death and liberation—depending on what happens). Phowa is a practice that can also be used to help others who are dying to have a peaceful and complete process. Most people, even most American Buddhists, are unfamiliar with it. I knew nothing about it when I first took the course. But I had been very impressed by the energy and magnetism of Ayang Rinpoche at a short teaching I attended in New York City in the fall of 2008. I was also convinced that the Tibetan Buddhists knew the "technology" for a good transition from death to rebirth.

In case you are wondering why I am standing firmly on the ground of rebirth (as opposed to the more common Western notion of a single birth and death), it is because I have become convinced of the validity of rebirth. That conviction has arisen from actual experiences I have had that do not include direct awareness of previous lives or knowledge of earlier periods of time. My experiences have come either within meditation practice or as a result of it. I have checked on them with several meditation masters and have come to embrace their validity. And even though I was not familiar with phowa in 2008, I had studied the map of the bardos between death and birth, with their confusing and overwhelming effects, as well as opportunities for liberation

within them. Phowa (through one's own efforts and/or the
assistance of a phowa master or even an experienced practitioner) can take one's consciousness into a state of clarity.
There, one may be fully liberated or choose wisely a next
life that can be most helpful to suffering beings and oneself
(the bodhisattva path). If none of this makes sense to you,
please forgive me. My experiences with phowa and Tibetan
teachings are a necessary part of my story; they are doors
that have opened as a result of losing Ed and becoming more
engaged in my direct experience.

Although I had been practicing Buddhism since 1971,
I had not studied any forms of Tibetan Buddhism. My
practices, first of Zen and then vipassana, were with Asian-
trained American Buddhist teachers. It may seem to you that
all Buddhist practices are exotic and a bit esoteric, but my
experience had been otherwise. Meditation and other practices made sense. Once I had some mastery, they gave me a
platform of compassionate optimism and skill from which
to embody my often-challenging life. By late 2008, I felt my
legs were under me, so to speak, when it came to Buddhist
meditation and dharma (teachings about the underlying
spiritual nature of our experience).

But at the Garrison Institute, I encountered unknown
territories. The powerful energetic field transmitted by
Ayang Rinpoche literally moved me. What I mean is that
my body moved wildly and involuntarily during many
practices and I experienced flashing internal colors and
"winds"—shaking energies—I had not previously encountered. When I met with Ayang Rinpoche privately during

the retreat, he told me I needed to take the phowa course in Bodh Gaya, India, so that I could find the full impact of the teachings. After some concern and anxiety about Rinpoche's invitation—for example, I was in terrible debt, my husband was scarily ill, and I didn't know where my life was going—I promised to attend the phowa course in Bodh Gaya "some day."

In late December 2012 and early January 2013, I am fulfilling that promise. To be perfectly clear, India never called to me and I was reluctant to go. But Ayang Rinpoche called to me. I could see that he was clearly not an ordinary mortal. Rinpoche broadcasts a signal, like a radio signal, picked up in my crown chakra, sending thrilling waves of energy moving through me, exciting my heart and filling me with vitality. And so, I was on my way to Bodh Gaya to be with Rinpoche again.

Just before we left New York City, I began to feel fatigue, aches and pains, and a sore throat. Even though I had had the flu shot, I could tell I was getting sick with something like a flu. As it turned out, I probably had "para-influenza virus," which causes flu-like symptoms but not fever. When we (I was traveling with a friend to meet up with other friends) reached Paris, where we rested for a couple of days before pushing on to Delhi, I hardly left my room. I slept for hours and didn't have much appetite. The worst of the aches and pains stopped and my symptoms changed to nasty sinus drainage and a persistent cough.

The flight from Paris to Delhi is about 9 hours and we arrived late at night. Once inside the international airport

I immediately notice the pale-blue smokiness of the atmosphere. This brings to mind an interview with Mira Nair, one of my favorite filmmakers, that I had read. She talked about how much she loved the ambience of her native India: the smoke, spices, incense, and pollution, all mixed together. With my now-irritated respiratory system and my fragile health, I just can't love the smoke.

I meet a charming young Indian woman in line at customs and we chat about the great spiritual opportunities of her country (she is in a doctoral program in psychology and spirituality at the University of Illinois). But I am more aware of the burning of my eyes and the endless annoying confusions, piled upon my anxieties, about how to exchange money and how to buy bottled water, sold only in machines for which we had no correct coinage. Nothing really works well or smoothly. After perhaps an hour and a half when we finally get outside the airport I am able to buy some water, but the vendor says, "I have no change," and charges me twice the price. Okay, I say to myself, "This is India"—my new mantra.

We are to spend a quick overnight at a "Western-style" hotel in Delhi, around 5 miles from the airport. Coming out of the airport, our transport van is stopped by military police and then after driving through what looks like a bombed-out exurban area, we are stopped again at the entrance of our hotel to be inspected by armed guards. This is India. By the time I get into my room, I feel quite paranoid. The place looks tawdry at 2:00 a.m. and I fear I might see rats scurrying across the floor. A friend, an American

Buddhist nun living in India, told me to rip apart the bedding to see if there are bedbugs before I accept any hotel room (she said I'd see the bloodstains on the mattress as a telltale sign). She also said to check the shower and the closets to see if they work. I am too tired to rip apart the bedding or inspect the hinges or the shower or the closet. The room has a Holiday Inn–wannabe feel to it. There is a flat-screen TV and a king-size bed with a duvet-type cover. But there is no hot water when I get into the shower. When I reach up to turn out the light next to my bed, the whole fixture crashes to the floor, leaving small shards all over the night table. This is India. I fall asleep after taking a small dose of Ativan (which I never take but had blessedly brought with me, just in case my supplement of melatonin didn't work).

I am not feeling good in my body or my surroundings when, early the next morning, I open the curtains to a bizarre-looking scene outside. There are *huge* fake-looking red "sofas" set up in a concrete courtyard around a shallow fake-looking swimming pool. Perhaps 20 to 25 youngish men meander around, carrying this and that. A few are climbing up a steel canopy, decorating it with gold and white nylon drapes. In a flash, I realize they are decorating for a wedding—a scene right out of Nair's *Monsoon Wedding*. I feel comforted by that thought. I arrive at the buffet breakfast, surrounded by an army of Indian businessmen all dressed in suits and carrying briefcases; now I know this is an "airport hotel" that principally houses corporate sojourners. I almost make the mistake of taking a piece of fruit from the buffet!

"Don't eat anything that is not peeled, sealed, or cooked—and make sure you peel it yourself!" Another mantra.

We arrive back at the Delhi airport to go through countless inspections of our tickets and boarding passes until we get up to the front of the security line and are told that the passes issued to us by Air France are "no good." In the meantime, an Australian friend, whom I have not seen for a year and a half, is waving and throwing me kisses from the other side of security. She's gotten through. Eventually we get our boarding passes and are allowed to the front of the security line. I had picked up Mary Karr's memoir *Lit* at JFK and am heavily into her rambling tale of boozing and downward spiraling. I haven't yet gotten to the part about her spiritual search. The mood created by Karr—with her extreme acting out and her desperation to get things right—sets a tone. Her shenanigans resonate with my emotional states (I am going a little crazy or maybe really crazy).

When we land at Gaya, in northern India near the Himalayas, the first thing I notice is the Tibetan-style architecture of the recently built airport. It is meant to appeal to spiritual pilgrims like me. The historical Buddha was enlightened nearby and now the area is populated by about 125 monasteries, many of them Tibetan. Hundreds of thousands of spiritual pilgrims visit here each year. As we step off the plane, I hear a familiar chant. The loudspeakers are playing the Buddhist refuge vows in Pali ("I take refuge in Buddha, dharma, sangha"), a language close to the Buddha's. I have many times taken these vows in retreats or ceremonies and now they are background Muzak! A huge golden

Buddha statue sits right in the middle of the airport teeming with Buddhist monks, nuns, and other practitioners. Buddhism is definitely the brand here.

In our taxi on the way out of the airport, at first the countryside looks serene. There are trees (never again to be seen) lining the road that leads into Bodh Gaya. I notice a few people tilling fields, but mostly my eye is attracted to feral dogs either sleeping or frolicking in fields. These dogs are unlike any wild dogs I have previously seen in Thailand (where they ran in packs and were skittish) or in South Africa (where they were skinny and miserable). These Indian dogs exude joy. Some are busily tending pups and others are playing together (not in packs, but as individuals) and still others are sleeping peacefully at the side of the road, relaxed about their safety. These dogs radiate life and curiosity and calm. This is India.

As we get closer to Bodh Gaya, the road becomes crowded and hectic. We are immersed into the chaos of this time of high spiritual pilgrimage when there are large retreats attended by people from all over the world, mostly from Asia. There is a constant assault on all my senses. Nothing is serene. In the road, I see hordes of people, cows, bulls, dogs, goats, and boars mixed with a barrage of motored vehicles and bicycle rickshaws. There are hundreds of formally dressed Buddhist monks and nuns—mostly in gold and maroon robes, the colors of Tibetan religious orders—and hundreds more ragtag Indians, some filthy and ill, carrying their loads on their heads or begging or pushing to get by. Horns and motorcycles and rickshaws blare the sounds of their machines (sometimes a little rap music, here and there) along with the human shouting and grunting and demanding. The mix of smoke, noxious pollution, nauseating sewage, sweet spices, and human sweat assaults the nose. The taste of sewage and various kinds of carbon fuels and occasional fried foods sticks to my taste buds. My body alternately feels hot, afraid, or exhausted as we bounce along with this jumble of life and death (once we saw a stiff long corpse, wrapped in a black blanket, being held by three people sitting in the backseat of an open-air Jeep). My mind is overwhelmed by the misery and chaos and then overwhelmed by stimulation and then uplifted by beautiful silver cows with calm pretty faces.

Inside a couple of days, we repeatedly brave the road into the main temple marketplace of Bodh Gaya, in motorized rickshaws with an oncoming flood of traffic and children that sluices off as we fly forward into the opposing flow. There are no traffic rules. You are hurtling yourself wildly into everything coming at you.

At the Mon Lam Retreat, thousands of mostly Tibetan monks and nuns, and other religious and lay Buddhists, gather to hear the teachings of the handsome fresh-faced 17th Kagyu Karmapa, the beloved spiritual leader of Tibet who is well known also in America and Europe. *Karmapa* means "embodiment of Buddha activities." Different from His Holiness the Dalai Lama, who is both a political and spiritual leader, the Karmapa is dedicated to spiritual teaching. Born in 1985 to a nomadic family and identified as the reincarnated 16th Karmapa when he was 7 years old, this

Karmapa is surprisingly practical and guileless. I was in his first audience in America on May 16, 2008, in New York City—with 5,000 other people. Once again, I am in a crowd of at least 5,000 under this huge tent except now at least 3,000 are Tibetan Buddhist monks and nuns—many of the monks being young boys. We've all been searched and scanned in order to get into the tent on the grounds of the Karmapa's monastery. His Holiness the Karmapa (HHK) makes his way into the tent with little ceremony.

Immediately he tells us he is suffering badly from the flu. He wasn't sure he could withstand the challenge of giving his talk. I am comforted by the fact that he speaks openly of his weakness. I have been feeling especially weak and white and fragile next to my brown brothers and sisters—Indian and Himalayan—who soldier on under conditions worse than I could have imagined. HHK says he is weak and yet he is happy that the teachings for 2013 have concluded in a satisfying way because too often, he says, obstacles interfere with his plans. He wonders why. And then he proceeds to give a clear and inspiring presentation about our attitude toward practice. He begins by saying that one can do prostrations and mantras "because you see others doing them" and they are perhaps of benefit—better than doing nothing. But the true attitude of practice is to investigate your experience and see what happens: If I do this practice, how does it benefit others and me? If I don't do this practice, what happens? In such a way, we become responsible for our daily practice with a sense of why we are doing it. We clarify our motivation. Until we have the direct awareness of why we engage in practices—meditation and others—we cannot get the full benefits they were designed to provide. He concludes by encouraging everyone to investigate their own experience in practice and to be honest and responsible about what we are doing. This is Bodh Gaya. I love it.

In the early evening, one of our two personal ambassadors to Bodh Gaya comes to meet us in our hotel lobby. Ayang Rinpoche has kindly assigned our group of four Westerners two assistants. One is an American woman (from Eugene, Oregon) in her mid-fifties who is an ordained *ani* or "nun" in Rinpoche's phowa lineage. She functions as a teacher of math and English for elementary school–age Tibetan monks (many begin their training at the age of 4 years and leave behind their families of origin). She lives mostly near Bangalore in southern India, where Ayang Rinpoche has his main monastery.

Now we are meeting our other ambassador, a 30-year-old cherub-faced young man who is at least 6 feet tall and has a beautiful white-toothed smile and golden skin. His name is Lama Y. We greet one another with bows and sit down for a chat in the lobby. When we ask Lama Y where he lives, he tells us he stays at a monastery in southern India. We ask him how he came to be a student of Rinpoche's. He went early in his life to the monastery. He's from an Indian family where he is one of 11 children and his parents were not happy about his leaving, but he wanted to go at the age of 4 years.

Lama Y asks if we would like to meet privately with

Ayang Rinpoche before the retreat begins? "Oh, yes," we reply enthusiastically. This is an honor. Lama Y checks by cell phone and reports that Rinpoche will see us right away! We hurry upstairs to get ourselves dressed and readied with the various gifts we are bringing. Then we pile into a motorized rickshaw and pour through the onslaught of Bodh Gaya at night. In one sharp turn, we narrowly miss hitting a toddler who is in a main intersection. Our vehicle is rushing us to the Vietnamese Buddhist temple where Ayang Rinpoche is staying during his sojourn in Bodh Gaya. The temple is elegant and quiet. We arrive in Rinpoche's room, heated by a propane space heater, to sit with him while we ask our questions and offer our gifts.

Rinpoche is a large man, more than 6 feet tall, with a broad open face. He is quiet, his eyes barely open, sitting on a bed. He moves subtly in and out of a meditative state. He talks little, but his presence is powerful. I ask if he is well because, like so many others in Bodh Gaya, he is coughing. Yes, he says, he is well. We ask a few questions about the retreat. I want only to be in his presence without speaking. Finally, he blesses us while placing traditional Tibetan *khatas* (white silk scarves symbolizing purity and compassion) on the backs of our necks, our heads bowed. Individually, he embraces our heads in his hands and chants a short prayer. We leave, thanking him. On the way back to our hotel, I love India. There is a disco-themed wedding going on in the hotel courtyard when we arrive and at first I am thrilled (once again, shades of *Monsoon Wedding*) and then I am up almost all night listening to Bollywood music played at a deafening volume. The next morning, I hate India and feel I am getting a new sore throat.

In the streets, we are always surrounded by the rush of life (along with the stench and everything else) and by thin and often very dirty children, ages 1 or 2 years through perhaps 12 or so. We give a rupee or two to many and give food when we can. Any food we have left over after eating is always carried to families and children. Through our guides, we find the Be Happy Cafe, run by a Canadian woman married to an Indian man. This café has water that is safe to drink, espresso drinks, coffee, Coca-Cola, and food selections called "pizza" and "spaghetti" (that vaguely measure up to their names) as well as flourless chocolate cake. In my imagination, I would have thought I should avoid eating in a place that panders to Westerners, but now, I want to eat only here. Each time we leave Be Happy, we have food to give to the small families living in shacks across the lane.

Just down the lane is a towering pile of plastic trash interlaced with food scraps. All the animals graze there: huge Brahmin bulls and elegant silver cows sleep on top of trash, alongside the grazing goats, dogs, and chickens. The bulls and cows look drunk with satiation. I never see any animal chase or attack another. The dogs don't fight or chase the chickens and the hairy boars don't push the goats out of the way. Once I saw a woman raise a broom to hit a dog that howled and screamed as though it had been beaten. Hearing him, dogs everywhere lifted their heads and pointy ears and began to run in his direction, saying, "Wait! What is happening to my friend?"

After the weather gets cold—dipping down to freezing—people burn plastic trash to keep warm, filling the air with toxic particulates. People also kindly put jackets and sweaters and burlap bags on the goats to keep them from shivering. Seeing a pink-nosed goat wearing a pink satin bed jacket following along behind a huge Brahmin bull is a hilarious treat. In scary traffic jams when we are stuck together like a mushed-up mess of life and machines, a cow or bull occasionally pushes you gently from behind if you are not moving fast enough, but the touch is friendly and easy, not threatening.

The schedule for our retreat says that on most of the 10 days we will begin at 7:00 a.m. It doesn't say exactly when the day will end. We have to rise at 5:30 a.m. to arrive on time. As it turns out, Ayang Rinpoche can sit on his meditation throne for 10 to 12 hours without getting off to eat or eliminate! He teaches (in both English and Tibetan), jokes with his assistants, chants, and meditates in a powerful silence with us, and then he blesses his followers with khatas and confers with those who want to meet him during the times we are on tea break or having lunch. He is remarkable and hearty, even though he is almost 80 years old. We cannot keep up with his energy. He reminds us repeatedly that our practices will work only if we have "pure motivation." What is pure motivation? It is selfless motivation to help the suffering beings. What is impure motivation? It is the desire to help only yourself or your family. He repeatedly warns against being motivated primarily to help your family and relatives. He ends each day when he believes his objectives have been fulfilled. Mostly this means participating for 10 to 12 hours of practice, much of it listening to teachings and some of it, meditating. There is no Q and A. In the first few days of the retreat, I am in contact with Rinpoche's energies and feel vitalized. Someone observing me says, "You were in a trance for hours." This is true of many at the retreat.

The mornings at first are cool, the days are warm, and the evenings are cool. Even though I am somewhat ill, I am feeling good. Then the weather changes and temperatures drop. In the afternoon, they fall to freezing or close to it. There is no heat in our meditation tent, with its 300 coughing participants (mostly Himalayan peoples from Tibet, Nepal, and Ladakh). To honor my small group of four, Rinpoche has asked us to sit in the front row, just in front of him. White and female and in the front row—wrapped and covered with whatever we can find, wearing surgical masks—we are highly visible.

Behind us sit the monks and nuns who have traveled from Australia, Canada, Vietnam, India, and Tibet. Most of them are brown people. Many are as old or older than we are. To my right is a Tibetan couple: long-time practitioners (the man has a scripture binder that is discolored and rumpled). Like the other Himalayan people, this couple is obviously poor, but they are sturdy, cheerful, and devoted. The Tibetans sit without moving for hours on end on the damp floor on a flat cushion in a cross-legged (not the lotus-style, but what we used to call "Indian-style") position with sagging backs and shoulders (although they straighten up during the meditations). Though they cough and sniffle, they do not seem exhausted. I sit upright in half-lotus and Japanese-kneeling posture. I get tired and have to shift my position too often (every half hour or so). Some Tibetan practitioners vibrate involuntarily with the flow of spiritual energy for most hours of the day (except for the tea breaks and meals); they are fully in trance states.

On the fourth day, I leave the retreat early with one of my friends (they are both sick with fever and flu). When we get back to our rooms, I foolishly eat some food that I have left in my room from the night before. I stupidly did not refrigerate it because I assumed that its having been cooked would preserve it even though it had cheese in it. The next morning I am violently sick with vomiting and diarrhea. In the early morning hours, I phone my other friends to say I am very ill, only to find that they also have decided to stay at the hotel: One is nauseated and the other has a fever and respiratory illness.

I sink back into my bed, trying not to vomit. Ayang Rinpoche appears to me in a vision: "You must return to the course," he says in a fierce tone. I reply in an equally fierce tone (not at all what would have been my manner in waking life), "I am too ill," with my arms folded over my chest. "You must return," he says simply, and I reply, "Make me well!" With that, I fall asleep. Over the next 5 or 6 hours I become so sick that I cannot stand up or straighten out my torso. I am bent over, my stomach in sharp pain. Dry heaves and nausea make it impossible for me to keep down any medicine or even Coca-Cola. I hang on to a simple mantra we are supposed to chant to Amitabha Buddha, but gradually

I realize that I am too weak to recover on my own. I ask a friend, an American doctor, to take me somewhere that will give me IV fluids.

At the front desk of the hotel, they tell him that a taxi will know where to take me for help. I get loaded into the backseat in a heap and the taxi makes its bumpy way through the flow of animals, humans, and machines. Finally we stop at something called "government clinic." When I hear the word "clinic," I feel relief—until I hobble inside where I spy a series of rooms in which scores of really sick people are lying on the floor in the darkened afternoon light; many are children. Someone escorts me into what looks like an office and I am asked what is wrong: diarrhea and vomiting. They don't ask my age, or to show my passport, but put me into a small room where an officious man tells me to lie down on a table covered with rubber. Someone mumbles "American" and puts a cloth cover on another table and says, "Move."

I am in a room with "windows" that are simply openings in the walls to the outdoors. The temperature is near freezing. I am wearing a light down vest over a lightweight fleece. I had never imagined there wouldn't be indoor heating. On the edge of my awareness, I notice a woman to my left about 10 feet away, the only other person on one of these tables. From the sound of it, she is having a baby—not her first because she is not making the painful cries of a first birth. I send her some blessing prayers. I cannot lift my head to see her. Another woman is helping her.

There are no doctors available here. A nurse or attendant comes to see me. My friend, the American doctor, says,

"I am a doctor. Can I help?" Without seeing any credentials from him, they allow him to help with getting the IV fluids and to give me a shot of an anti-nausea drug. For at least 2 hours, a political rally takes place in an adjacent room that is perhaps 20 feet away from me. A man screams through a megaphone and about 60 people listen and shout back. Someone puts a wool blanket over me, and my friend asks for a second (I am shivering). The response: "One blanket, one person. Government rule." The taxi driver from the hotel offers to go back and get another blanket. That shames the attendant into giving me another. Even on the IV and with the anti-nausea drug in my system, I am very ill; I retain just enough awareness to recite the prayer to Amitabha Buddha for those around me and myself. I begin to surrender myself and to wonder if I will die here. After all, I have come to Bodh Gaya because Ed is ill and dying and because Richard is ill and dying and because I myself will be dying soon. Perhaps I have come to die.

At that very moment, the drugs and IV fluids seem to kick in and I feel more relaxed. The woman on the next table brings her new baby, wrapped lightly in her sari, to show my friend and me. Two nights before, on our way back from the retreat, it so happened that my American friend noticed a small storefront clinic run by a medical doctor, Dr. K, and stopped to have a conversation with him. Now it turns out that Dr. K visits the clinic a couple of times a day. When he sees me—who had been healthy a couple of days ago— he says, "What happened to you?" My friend goes out to Dr. K's clinic to see if it is possible to obtain some medicine for me there that would allow me to go back to my heated hotel room.

While my friend is gone, I hear the young mother speaking sweetly to her newborn while she suckles it. Then an old woman (her mother?) arrives and begins to burn something I assume is incense. Soon, though, the room is filled with blue smoke. I lift my head to see the old woman sitting next to the baby and mother, burning what seems to be a bonfire in a metal container on the table. Part of the fire falls to the floor and is burning there like the fires in the street. Ah, I think calmly, now I will die in the fire. I cannot get up. I am too weak and I don't know where I am. The blue smoke thickens to a threatening level, just as my friend and a nurse arrive in the room. They are shocked. The nurse screams at the old woman and makes her leave; she takes her fire—in a large pan—with her. She continues to burn it in the anteroom where the political rally ended hours before. My friend tells me he has medicines that can work without the IV, and I am unhooked from it and walk unstably out of the clinic into the cold night where trash fires are burning everywhere. We take a taxi back to the hotel and I fall into bed. I take some anti-nausea medication that I am able to keep down with Coca-Cola and I fall into a stupor-like sleep.

The next day I am well enough to read but not to return to the retreat. I read the only book I brought from home (I had finished *Lit* by Mary Karr)—*Hunger Mountain: A Field Guide to Mind and Landscape*. This book connects the mountain I see every day, Hunger Mountain of the

Worcester Range of the Green Mountains, with 5th- and 6th-century Chinese ideographic poems. The book teaches about the space between things and the ways that nature reveals impermanence. It is written by David Hinton, an acclaimed translator of ancient Chinese works, who lives about 5 miles up the road from me. I have hiked Hunger Mountain many times, and Hinton writes meditations on the landscape there. Reading, I sink back into my identity with Vermont, my profession of psychotherapy, my friendly American Buddhist sangha, the quiet serenity of my Vermont surroundings that support me, the care I give to Ed and Richard, and the gratitude I feel for my American doctor friend who saved my life. I perceive a complete crystalline beauty in my particular existence. I don't need to search any further, even if I never perfect my practice of phowa. I now have links to Ayang Rinpoche's community and surely someone will help my friends and me as we are dying. I don't have to do it all myself.

When I return to the phowa course, a little shakier and thinner than when I left, the hardy Himalayan people are soldiering on; the shakers are still shaking; the couple next to me are sicker, but holding firm in their dedication. Rinpoche is steaming toward the conclusion of the retreat.

The final day I attend, I last only until 8:00 p.m. At this point, Rinpoche is shepherding our group to the Mahabodhi Temple to chant under the famed Bodhi tree—a relative of the banyan tree under which the Buddha was enlightened about 2,600 years ago. Because of my illness, I have not yet visited the Bodhi tree. I tried once, but leaving my rubber boots in the public place provided for them—you must remove your shoes to enter—was a tricky proposition. It would have been "Bye-bye, boots!" Now I am prepared with a bag in which to carry my boots. It is dark and we are going to chant by candlelight. But I am the only member of our small group who wants to go to the temple; the others want to go back to our hotel to rest. I am still sick and weak. My friends convince me not to stretch my luck. I go back to the hotel and the next day we leave for Paris to return to Vermont. Remarkably, I return home without having visited the most important Buddhist pilgrimage site in the world: the Bodhi tree of Bodh Gaya.

I don't regret this final decision. It is in alignment with what I have learned on this particular extension of my love pilgrimage: that I am complete as I am and in the love I give and get. I go out to see Ed at his care center as soon as I am able. I have been away for a month. Ed has regressed a lot. He has become wholly incontinent in both his bladder and bowel functioning. The staff tells me that he seemed okay for the first couple of weeks, but then it was as though his entire body noticed my absence and he became more and more infantile. Of course, in seeing me, he is overjoyed and seems even to understand that I have brought him some simple gifts from India—a Tibetan *thangka* and a small statue of a sleeping Buddha. When I tell him that I have been to India where the Buddha was enlightened, he is thrilled and says he is very happy for me. It is obvious that Ed knows I exist in a world wholly apart from his. There is something fully acknowledged between us now that I have returned from what has been an exotic and treacherous journey: I am in a world entirely separate from him. This separation no longer saddens me, not even a whit. I have released Ed many times and now I have released myself as well. I am in a new life.

In this way and that I tried to save the old pail

Since the bamboo strip was weakening and about to break

Until at last the bottom fell out.

No more water in the pail!

No more moon in the water!

—Mugai Nyodai in *Zen Flesh, Zen Bones*

7.

At the end of the summer of 2013, I spend a lot of my free time on my favorite pond—locally dubbed #10 Pond—in my yellow two-person pedal boat. With my new beau, Robert, and my new dog, Peony, I tour the 10-acre pond (a glacial lake from the last ice age) and learn new things. This summer I am astonished to see a bald eagle couple nesting high in a pine on the east side of the pond, the shores of which are fully protected from real estate development. Sometimes I also spot the male eagle soaring and swooping. There is an eagle offspring in that nest, according to a stranger who swims up to the rock on the far shore where Robert and I stop to sunbathe today. The stranger says that a parent eagle snatched a baby loon or egg to feed the baby eagle at the start of the summer and that is why there is only one young loon, instead of the typical two, this year. This is shocking news—not because of the brutality of the event itself—because I could not have imagined it. The pond teaches me something new in almost every visit, every 2 days or so, all summer long.

Until I got my yellow pedal boat 3 months ago, I would swim out from a little drop-off from the dirt road that follows the west shore, pretending I was the poet Mary Oliver, submerging myself carefully into "my" Black Pond (black at night and in some spots during the day; it is 130 feet deep). I named the drop-off "Polly's Beach." Now I pedal anywhere I want to go on the pond and swim off rocks. And my boat, due to the kindness of a generous man, lives on the shore of #10.

In my day job, I still sit across from therapy clients or supervisees for 35 to 40 hours per week and I still go out to give talks at conferences and organizations. You might find it hard to believe how much I enjoy these things. I am always amazed by what I learn from those I meet through my work. Over the years since Ed's diagnosis, I embrace the proposition that "the road comes up to meet me." In other words, I am interested and often fascinated with what comes to me, including the people who sit with me in my consulting room. That doesn't preclude my planning and having wishes and desires. Notably, I look especially closely at what arises in the face of my own plans and desires. Things rarely go as I imagine they will or should. Sometimes they fall apart in a painful but fascinating way.

For example, about 2 weeks ago, I was having the traditional Saturday dinner at the Bee's Knees with Ed and

Richard; it was a luminous warm sunny evening and we were seated outside on the patio where I leashed Peony to my chair. Richard and I are conversing and Ed is staring at passersby. There is a celebratory mood because the table service is good, the weather is warm, and the dog is enjoying bits of food that I drop for her (creating bad-dog begging). At the end of our meal (which is not a stellar feast, but good enough), a van pulls up in front of the restaurant and the band that will be playing later starts unloading its equipment.

After I pay the check, I work hard to get Ed to understand that I want him to "stand up" and then to "step out" into a narrow space. Peony is pulling on the other end of her leash and Richard has toddled off on his cane toward my car. My iPad is tucked under my arm. Ed is having a hard time with balance. I am distracted by the dog and by Ed's struggle. In a flash, I look up and see that Richard has climbed into the band's van and taken a seat. "NO, Richard!" I yell and raise my left arm to gesture to him, releasing my iPad to drop edge-first across my left toes. "Shit!" I scream. Neither Ed nor Richard has any capacity to pay attention to my pain. Neither looks in my direction as I collapse down over my foot, worried I may have broken a toe. My third toe hurts a lot. When I glance up at Ed, he looks bewildered and scared. I pop right up even though I am in considerable pain. Richard is climbing out of the van, saying, "That's not our car," with a big grin on his face. I let go of Ed and hobble over to unlock my car and help Richard get into the backseat. I open the back hatch and Peony lunges in, certain we are in an emergency because she picks up on my anxiety and pain. By now Ed has wandered over to the little fence at the periphery of the patio and is peering in my direction like a lost child, afraid he cannot get out of the enclosure. I go back to him. We get as far as the front door of my car, moving very slowly. He is wobbly and confused. The car door is open, but Ed cannot determine what is next. I try to guide him by telling him, "Just bend down," and then I show him, but he is too afraid and confused. Richard shouts from the backseat, "Just get IN the car, Ed!"

A man from the band, who looks like he's in his late forties, shows up at the curb: "Do you need some help?" I see the future: Ed will soon not be able to get into any car. I cannot push him down or make him bend. This man tries to encourage Ed to stoop over. Ed is staring straight into the man's face as if to say, "WHO in the HELL are YOU?" The man responds by saying, "Maybe I am just making things worse," and I tell Ed, "You don't know him. He is helping out. Just get into the car." I ask the man to stay with me. I have visions of having to call an ambulance to get Ed to move.

Then the man and I have the same idea: pull the car out farther from the curb so that Ed has plenty of room to walk in the street over to the opening. The man holds on to Ed and I close the door and move the car. I explain to Richard that Ed can't get into the car because he's forgotten how to do it. After the car is far enough away from the curb, the other man and I are able to get Ed to move into it. Phew. I thank the stranger and drive off, shaken, but relieved that we are all safe now. My left foot is killing me. I tune in to

A Prairie Home Companion on the radio. Then I replay the entire scene in my mind's eye and laugh at the hilarity of it all. Richard thinks I am laughing at the radio show and Ed doesn't think at all. Life has come up to meet me in ways that I hadn't imagined: the van, Richard's confusion, the sore toes, the help in getting Ed into the car, and the preview of things to come.

When I arrive back home, almost 2 hours later, I tell my friend Robert about what happened and he immediately laughs hard. I ice my foot and take an Advil. You might be wondering about Robert. Writing this book has given me an important opportunity to tell my story of loss freely in my own words. You probably know that you need to tell your story (even repeatedly) after a serious loss or trauma, but (as I said earlier) I became guarded about telling my story in the midst of stereotypes about Alzheimer's, grief, marriage, and love. When you are forced by life to change your identity and circumstances, you eventually need to shift away from a story of loss and write a whole new story of life.

What does it take to feel your life as precious after tragedy? I wanted to take my love for Ed forward and continue to live it in a new form in a new relationship. That is really where my new story began: I found myself confronted with the question of what love is and why I wanted it so much. I went all the way to Africa to begin to find out. Trying to discern what love is, while searching for it in my personal life, I developed a brave attitude of feeling through a lot of uncertainty and anxiety and seeing how the road comes up to meet me in the midst of it.

After my relationship with Deon ended, I began a series of phone conversations with a man my age who lives in California, someone I had known casually in the past. I was happy to talk to him because I didn't want to go out and "date" strangers, and so I spent a number of months getting to know a man who lives a mere 3,000 miles away. He called me every Monday night around 9:00, Eastern Standard Time. He knew Ed and me in the past, and he and I were familiar with each other through the Buddhist world. There was no exchange of daily e-mails, but we traded favorite poems and I saw him for several in-person visits. The relationship ended painfully. I moped around about it for several months vowing *not* to date, but still not wanting to live alone for the remainder of my life. Then I visited my daughter, Amber, and grandson, Clive, in LA over the Christmas holidays.

Amber is a powerhouse. She is a therapist and clinical supervisor at a clinic that helps kids and their families to get out of gangs and get their lives back on track. She heads up three therapeutic clinics in schools. I have become a great admirer of Amber, whom I would admire even if I were not her mother. She is a straight thinker, a straight shooter, an able and dedicated transformer of tough and hopeless young people—*and* she has a great sense of humor and her own style. Still, we can also be at odds. She totally rejects my moping. "He acted badly, Mom, and you just need to move on." As a result of such "support" from my daughter and some advice from a wise woman Buddhist priest friend who is a lot like my daughter ("Stop that moping around and go on a Web site; you aren't getting any younger"), I finally turn to an Internet dating service: a Web site—awkwardly called The Right Stuff—for people who attended or taught at an elite college or university. Although it sounds silly, the method works. I write a transparent description of myself and meet up with a few guys from New York and California. (I didn't want to look at locations too close to home because I like my privacy!)

In the fall of 2011, I meet Robert in New York City. Five years older than me, he is a psychiatrist, psychoanalyst, and author. Robert is divorced with a couple of grown daughters. We are compatible in our politics and personal styles. He has a refined intelligence and a sharp wit. He is an accomplished writer and embraces adventure in his personal life. I begin our first telephone conversation—as I did with everyone who made it that far into the inquiry—explaining my "special circumstances": I take care of two demented men who were my husbands. One was the "love of my life" and the other is the father of my children. My situation is unique. Most of the men I speak with have never heard of anything like it before—and either it makes sense to them or it does not. Robert is more than just accommodating; he is interested, maybe a little amused. On our first "date" in Vermont (I had met up with him once before in New York City to go to a play and dinner), we have dinner at the Bee's Knees with Ed and Richard. Robert takes it well. He claims my devotion is a sign of my loyalty and a good omen for him (in case he has to spend his last years in my care).

Almost 2 years later now, Robert still laughs at my predicaments and sees the bigger picture of the sacrifices involved. He has become my best friend and true witness. He praises and supports me even though we also bicker. He helps with Ed and Richard. Once he took Ed to the hospital emergency room during a snowstorm when I couldn't get out. Often he joins us at the Bee's Knees and accompanies me on the long car trips to and from the care centers—especially when the weather is treacherous.

When I am with Ed, I am still "Ed's wife" in the sense that I hug and kiss Ed and tell him I love him. I sit next to Ed and hold his hand or rub his back. Ed needs this kind of cherishment and I want to give it. Robert is more than tolerant about all this; he is caring and understanding. Naturally, Ed just accepts Robert as another person who is in our "family," typically assuming Robert is visiting him. Richard knows that I have a personal relationship with Robert and greets him warmly, "Hey, Bob, how are you?"

This is the way the road has come up to meet me: first, Ed in care outside my home and second, I have a new relationship. Because Ed is in care, I am able to have a separate life and to enjoy him when I see him. I want to tell others (especially those who have spouses with dementia) that residential care centers—as distinct from "nursing homes"—are places where people thrive when they cannot thrive at home. They don't go there "to die," in most cases, but "to live" in conditions they need. Residents get support and care that ease their anxiety and increase their joy and pleasure. Of course, residents also need family members to oversee their care. If family members have their own lives, they can readily provide what their dear ones need without resentment. I am deeply grateful for our residential care centers. The tragic disease of Ed's life did not cut down two lives; it cut down only one. Ed went into care before I collapsed and while he still had some essence of his personality available and could get to know and be known by other residents and staff. Many of the residents now look after Ed and ask after him when they see me. Richard's going into care has also released him to be the kind of gentleman he could never have been in the dangerous mess of hoarding and paranoia that accumulated around him during his last decade in St. Louis. Richard is far more relaxed and warm than I have ever known him to be and it has been a pleasure to get to know him in these last years. And now he has his girlfriend, who makes it easier for him to feel at home.

After Ed adjusted to living in care (after about only 2 weeks), his face brightened and my mood lifted because keeping him at home for the year and a half after he retired was a burden on both of us. Ed was listless, depressed, and confused. He couldn't organize himself without my help or help from someone else. I didn't know how much to feed him and he couldn't seek any food for himself. Before he went into care, he'd lost so much weight that I wondered if he was suffering from a metabolic disorder. In those first 6 months after Ed moved, I slept 8 to 10 hours every night to recover from the mental exhaustion that was the result of being constantly shadowed, mimicked, and needed. Ed initially objected to moving into care and I felt afraid about him going (both of these are typically present in a patient and a caregiver), but I knew the move was a necessary development for both of us. Even the divorce—which had to occur so that he could qualify for Medicaid—seemed right to me at the deepest level of my being. Ed could no longer be my husband.

August 3, 2008

I said something to Ed this morning and he said, "Why are you so hostile?" I said, "Hostile? I am not hostile." He replied, "You seem angry underneath. Is it because of the finances?" I said it was true that I had resentments and some of them had to do with finances and the pressures on me to pay down his credit cards. But I said that my anger had more to do with two other issues.

Ed wanted to know about them. I replied that (1) He doesn't treat me like a person with "subjectivity"— thoughts and feelings and life experiences. Rather, he tends to treat me like a piece of furniture that he uses and needs and moves around. I am worn down even though Ed is affectionate and wants to help me. I said I know when I am treated like a person and when I am not. And (2) Ed has used a dishonest "smoke and mirrors" approach to the big challenges or conflicts between us over the past 5 years or so. I find it difficult to see the truth of what he is doing. These themes, I said, have existed in the past between us— recalling how he'd deceived me financially prior to 5 years ago—but they are worse now. Ed seemed to grasp all this at some level.

Then I said that I was breaking away from him. I promised to care for him and love him always. I told him he was the "love of my life and my best friend" and that I would never abandon him in any way. However, I needed to have my own life, too. I elaborated that I was trying to "clear up some karmic bond" between us that kept us "entangled in an unwholesome way" and seemed to lead to his not having to look at the truth. He nodded.

I reminded him then that while I would care for him and protect him over the coming years, he could not do the same for me. I would have to care for and protect myself. I said, "I want you to understand that my life will become independent of you; it is independent now because I cannot depend on you." He seemed to understand.

I am endlessly thankful to the people who provide Ed's everyday care. They go beyond their duty to make him comfortable and at home. Can you imagine changing the diapers—several times a day—of someone who weighs about 200 pounds and thinks like a 1-year-old? It is demanding and upsetting for the staff just as it is for Ed. And finally, the staff and residents always acknowledge the vast love between Ed and me. They are witnesses. They celebrate our love. They are also unsurprised to see Robert sometimes accompanying me. They welcome him and say to me, "You need to have a life of your own."

Am I on the frontiers of human love to see "family" and "spouse" and "children" as categories that are flexible and changing and impermanent? I hold no conventional norms about who is on the inside and who is on the outside. My extended blended family of adulthood (which includes ex-husbands and my wife-in-law) has "worked" better for me than my nuclear family of childhood did. There are rifts and squabbles in our family, but generally they work out over time. The emotional weather in my childhood home was almost always threatening or stormy. I have had better emotional weather in my blended family.

I truly enjoy the company of my adult son, Colin, and his wife, Melissa, just as I enjoy the company of Amber (who is happily divorced) and Clive. I also enjoy Arne (Richard's first child) and his wife, Sarah, and son, Finn. Colin and Melissa live in Ottawa, Ontario, and Arne and Sarah live near Toronto, Ontario. Part of my family is Canadian! I am not as close to Ed's son, Noah, and his wife, Rachel, and their two children, Izzy and Will, but I wish them well and am happy they are thriving. Our children have all done very well in their adult lives: They are responsible citizens, are caring partners and parents, with meaningful and dedicated careers. I continue to rely on my wife-in-law and her husband for support and help in times of family crisis. Colin and Melissa have frequently lent their help and services in supporting me in helping Ed. Richard's three children share the tasks of being his power of attorney and paying his bills.

I define "family" as a group of people who care about one another's needs and happiness and do what is possible to provide for them. They may also be witnesses to one another; some may love one another, but it is not necessary that everyone love everyone else—only that they respect one another and care about one another's welfare. These people may or may not have any biological ties. When such a caring group exists, it is a problem-solving unit—a messy problem-solving unit. That means that when a crisis or difficulty arises, the individuals know where to turn in order to get help. It does not necessarily mean that the help arrives smoothly or in all the best packages but only that the individuals keep trying to solve the problems.

It might be important to have a "family story"—such a story helps people identify themselves with a group or a tribe—but when the shit hits the fan, family must be more than a narrative. It must be a way of getting and giving help and seeing what is needed. My family life has never been stable, secure, or easy. Most people I know find the same conditions in their families—unpredictability, conflict, and strife—alongside whatever they can enjoy together. We may wish that family could be a haven, but family is not a haven, at least not after childhood is over. The sooner we learn that, the easier it is to look at things realistically. We need to find our havens elsewhere (in our spiritual practices, nature, partners, creativity, service, friends, dedication).

And yet, if you want to love in an active way, you should try to unfold and uncover what it means to be a reliable witness, a giver without resentment, a loyal friend in your messy family. Most parents do a good-enough job as parents if they can strike down the scaffolds of idealization of themselves, their children, and their family's status or reputation. In our family, those scaffolds were struck down for us and we continued to solve our problems and sustain our relationships. Not all families are that lucky; sometimes, the burdens of solving problems and working out relationships are just too great. When people ask me, as they sometimes do, "Why is it so hard for us to achieve world peace?" I respond by saying, "How are things going in your family?" Ordinary families include a lot of struggle, competition, jealousy, and even hatred in a way that mimics the conflict of nations.

Real families—not idealized fantasy families—have suffered and struggled and transformed their views of one another. These families have pockets of love. Some of the grown children get to know their parents as individuals, some parents see their children as three-dimensional real people with strengths and weaknesses, and some partners become best friends. Love is a demanding activity that takes mindfulness, attention, empathy, interest, and perseverance. In order for it to be a two-way street, both people have to be vulnerable and open. Even cherishment—love on a one-way street— is difficult, because in order to cherish another person, you have to be a careful witness and a thoughtful caregiver, as well as an enthusiastic friend.

Before I met Robert, my only true love story was a fated one: Ed was a stranger who said, "Oh, THERE you are!" The blueprint for my life with Ed came not from my plans and wishes, but from an unknown mysterious force. Although that has its wonders, it is not the only path to loving and being loved. Robert and I have a different story: I met him on a Web site. He was a stranger I got to know awkwardly at first. There was no overdetermined golden glow around his head. Gradually, I have come to say, "Oh, THERE you are, Robert!" My love for Robert is like a spring rain, drenching me slowly, almost imperceptibly. By nature, Robert is quiet and emotionally reserved; his humor tends to move along a continuum from the ironic to the sardonic. He is never hysterical or very expressive, but he is kind and patient and articulate—when he gets around to saying something. I investigate him in sideway glances even though we sometimes have intense and even combative arguments about (what else?) psychoanalytic theory and clinical technique.

We are old—or oldish—and know the freedom and exhilaration of *not* having to make a family together, share a life story, make our fortunes together, or worry too much about our children. (We do, however, care about the circumstances and news of each other's grown-up children.) In this expansive light, we can be gently curious as though we were sorting through old photographs (not digital images) and looking at them one at a time. We stare into each other's memories and ask about the details of when, where, what—what were you wearing, what was she wearing. There are countless stories like this about the rising and passing away of love affairs, family, real estate, travels, and accomplishments. I often revel in the slowness of sorting out these details even though I am possibly the most impatient person on earth.

On Sunday afternoon (what a golden time of the week!), we may watch a movie, share a pizza, and then talk about the details of what we think and feel, and why and where we learned them. Many mornings, before we go to yoga or work, I sit with Robert at our local Post Office Café in the tiny town of Worcester where I live, and I listen to him talk with local people. This morning he chatted with someone whose sister went to college with Robert at Reed College in Oregon! Suddenly, Robert is recalling names and life situations of people he and this fellow's sister knew in common. The sister now lives in Scotland and seems to have had an adventurous and expansive life, just like Robert. The process of seeing and being seen by Robert is a slow and rich unfolding with some surprising reflections through his widened blue eyes when he "sees" me in a way he's never done before—or when I search for myself there.

This is the way my life comes up to meet me as I come to love Robert. Some of my friends and colleagues seem anxious or even frightened by aging and diminishment, but Robert and I don't roll that way. Robert's childhood smells to me like it was "normal" or "regular" in a way that mine was not. Perhaps that allows Robert to trust that his life will rise up to meet him in his new home in Vermont—a place he'd not known much about before he came to know me. Robert says he still sometimes prefers the urbane excitement of New York City to the serene beauty of our mountain residence. All the same, he is willing to go forward without a lot of fuss about planning and "future." We both keep a close watch on the road in front of us.

Many aging clients come to therapy with a nervous sense about whether or not they "have enough money" or "have made the best plans" or "will be able to be happy" in their final years. Of course, it makes sense to have a general overview of what you want to do as you close down your existence on earth, but it is also important to pay close attention to what comes up to meet you. You've spent a lot of time in the business of your life once you are 5 or 6 decades into it, and you might just want to loosen your fantasy of control, at least a little. Just as Carl Jung sensed a "solidity underlying all existence and a continuity" in his way of being, you may begin to see, if you look clearly and acknowledge honestly the circumstances of your life, that you have not been in control of many of your discoveries and successes. They simply came to you from an unknown source.

Loving Ed has made this source explicit in my life. And loving Robert, I see it from a different angle. Robert doesn't fill up his time with distractions or anything else that takes him away from his appreciation of what he enjoys. It is Robert's goal to witness the beauty he sees here in the country, and there in the city, and in the people around him. Jung says, "The world into which we are born is brutal and cruel, and at the same time of divine beauty" and Robert agrees. Beauty—especially the natural beauty around us—draws Robert into deeper contact with me. I am proud and pleased with how he inhabits our relationship in these surroundings he never imagined. When you are facing a destabilizing or dispiriting situation, look straight into your experience, without freaking out, and you may see your own version of divine beauty and a mysterious foundation. There will be exhilaration right next to fear.

When I met with Eleanor Johnson—a videographer and filmmaker whose apartment is also her studio in New York City—to talk about love, we sat down at her place with a pot of coffee and French patisseries from a local bakery. Eleanor is my age, a Buddhist practitioner, and an accomplished artist. With her straight-cut dark hair and her all-black outfits, Eleanor looks mysterious. You just assume she is "somebody." We are good friends. Eleanor has taught me so much about living on the edge. In the past decade or so, she's had a hard time getting funding for her work and yet, she has continued to move forward and develop her vision through multiple film and video projects. At the start of our conversation, Eleanor declares, "There is a gift underpinning actualized love: It is a mutuality with the beloved if you have the humility to receive it. When you hold out your begging bowl, what is put into it has to be used and cared for. It has to be bigger than your self." At the end of our lives, we all hold out our begging bowls. We are no longer at the top of our game. Whatever is put into that bowl is what we need to engage with, what we must find meaningful and fascinating.

Eleanor tells me that she "had a wonderful long marriage to Judah, an Israeli. He was kind and tried hard to know me and see me. We tried to remain flexible in the face of challenges and to exchange self for other." But then this true love broke apart and "our lives were messed up. When my marriage ended, there was a tremendous loss, but also it was a gateway for me to develop. When you hurt that badly and break apart, what are you going to do? I had to take back everything I had projected into him and find it in myself. I was married for twenty years and now I am divorced for twenty-one. I had felt Judah to be more worthwhile and important than me. When our marriage broke up, I had to reassemble my self from the broken shards of the mirror." And this has been the heart of Eleanor's artistic development ever since. In one of her projects, she has people sit directly, face-first, in front of her camera and then she films them and asks questions about their own spiritual development. Afterward, she sits with them and shows them the film and they talk about it. In this way, she offers a powerful mirror that reveals their spiritual autobiography.

Eleanor believes that we are entering an era in which people in general will appreciate more deeply the spiritual path of love—partnership, friendship, and personal relationship. "My friend Bruce Chilton told me about the relationship between Mary Magdalene and Jesus: It was a personal relationship that was profound and transformative. There is still tremendous difficulty in family life and tremendous fear of dying, but I believe something is on the horizon— a new model based on the kind of relationship that Mary Magdalene and Jesus expressed: a love in which every man or woman can interpret another's experience through his or her own. This can become, as Thoreau has said, an opportunity to teach best what one needs to learn." Eleanor has a grand expansive vision—in her life and her work—and I don't always grasp the particulars of it, but I think she is talking about the mutual witnessing through vulnerability, conflict, need, and care that true love is.

I don't know if a new wisdom is developing on this score or not, but I do know that I have learned a whole new way of being as a result of loving Ed and losing him. So much was snatched away. As I let go of my belief that I controlled what was going to happen next, I came to know that I had not controlled it from the start. With the help of my spiritual teachers and Buddhist practices, my courage and confidence grew. I learned to talk to myself out loud and to laugh at myself out loud. I also learned to talk to the dog. The more I was alone, the more I felt accompanied after I started to pay attention. I discovered I was not alone but was supported by an awake and tender wisdom that is not my own.

Learning to love Robert within these complex circumstances has taught me to let go again and again of my own expectations, but not my needs. My needs bring up feelings and I am now pretty good at discerning the package of needs and feelings. Simply feeling my feelings—without necessarily speaking them or acting upon them—I have become more skillful in loving and being loved. I can now experience my needs with tenderness toward myself. I am rarely a critic of any need. I inquire into my own mind about what I would like to do about this need in relation to what is possible. Nothing is left out, but nothing is urgent.

This way of loving has also allowed me to love my grown children and their children in a new way. I feel fully present and deeply trusting even through our conflicts. Because I care terribly much about what happens to my children, in the past I often felt trapped in my needs for their happiness and my judgments about how they could reach that happiness. Now instead of feeling trapped, I have a trust and confidence in them to allow them fully their own mistakes, failures, and fears, and to see them, in this way, as a part of humanity. More important, I have noticed that same foundation under my children's being as I have found under my own. They are good people and their intentions and actions are generally infused with their ideals and skills, but they are not in control of their lives. They cannot guarantee that they will be happy, wise, or safe. And yet, I feel within them a wise mind that undergirds their efforts. Witnessing this has allowed me to hear about their pain, sorrow, and fear more fully.

Letting go and letting the bottom fall out (as it must) is the only way to love fully and truly. When love is on a two-way street, the stakes feel very high, and the bottom is likely to drop out sooner. The kind of love I have been extolling does not lead to greater calm, serenity, peace, or purity, at least not for me. Instead, it leads to greater freedom, the acceptance of loss, more confidence, and an always growing interest in what is rising up to meet you in living and dying.

Epilogue

I am writing this in late February 2014. Life continues in many ways as it has for the past 5 years, since Ed has been in residential care. And yet, there are also significant changes. Just as I had anticipated last summer, by late fall Ed could no longer get into a car, so I could no longer take him and Richard out for Saturday at the Bee's Knees. Naturally, this change has brought a bit of sadness for us all. Our Saturday outings were expansive and adventurous for Ed, Richard, and me (and even for Peony). Gone, too, are the Wednesday evenings out when Ed and I would go for pizza or a simple meal at the Craftsbury General Store.

Now I visit Ed at his care center on Wednesday evenings and take a few cookies or some candy so that I have something to share with him. This Wednesday, when I arrived at 6:30, I found that an aide had placed him on the sofa in the TV room. You have to move Ed very deliberately. He cannot rise from a chair on his own. Some kind of visceral instability makes it hard for him to stand up and get out of a chair and almost terrifying to lower himself into one. And so, he doesn't move unless someone pulls him up and escorts him to his next seat. He has grown very weak, perhaps from the effects of his disease or perhaps from sitting too much.

When I walk into the TV room and appear right in front of him (Ed never sees people coming and going; he is not able to follow things with his eyes), Ed looks shocked. He seems both thrilled and embarrassed. I give him hugs and kisses and sit down next to him. Three other residents greet me, happy to see Ed and me together again. In the background, on the TV news, the Winter Olympics are winding down and Kiev is burning. Perhaps because of the noise and the excitement, Ed seems unable to recognize me. I say, "I'm Polly," and he shakes his head in frustration as if to say, "Oh, of course. I knew that! I am so distressed not to be able to greet you by name!" At least that's how I interpret it. We share cookies and I watch some TV news. After a while, I pull Ed off the couch and we walk extremely slowly back to his room. He stares at me instead of watching the floor to see where he is going. When we get back to his room, I water his plant and talk to him. I turn on a music box and sit a little longer with him. Then I bend over and hug and kiss him, saying, "I love you, Ed!" He has not spoken a word to me during this visit. I leave, blowing him kisses as I go out the door.

On Saturday, I drive out to pick up Richard from his

care center. I haven't seen him since Valentine's Day—for which I brought him a card and candy, but more important, I also brought some candy and a card he could give to his sweetie. He was thrilled with that. Richard comes out of his center on his own (with the use of a cane) and easily gets into my car and gives me a hug. This is the first time I have not had to go into the center to get him! He must have been watching for me and feeling independent. Oddly, Richard's functioning still seems to be improving as Ed's is tragically declining. I wonder if this uptake in spirit is due to Richard's relationship. "It's supportive of your health to have someone to love," I say to myself. Richard says he's been feeling good and he comments on the spring-like temperatures and the beauty of this late winter day. Together we listen to Radiolab—an episode about death.

When we arrive at Ed's place, Richard steps out of the car onto the icy sidewalk and makes his way independently over to the front door. I have to get Peony out of the car and gather up a few things. By the time Peony and I are inside, Richard has toddled off down the hallway to Ed's room. He's the first to get in and I hear him greeting Ed enthusiastically. "Hey, Ed, it's Richard! How are you?" Peony precedes me into the room, and by the time I see Ed, he is looking a little terrified. For him, it must seem that all of these multiple things have suddenly come out of nothing. Ed is staring at Richard as if to say, "Who are YOU?" and he even looks at Peony with confusion. When we are all finally seated and Peony's orange winter coat has been removed, Ed seems to recall who we are. He is delighted to see us. He adores stroking and petting Peony, and she adores receiving his endless attention.

Richard and I try to talk with Ed a little, especially to tell him who we are. Ed seems to get it. Then I ask Richard if he wants to look up anyone on Google because I have my iPad with me. Sometimes we look up performers, songs, and shows from the seventies, eighties, and nineties (for example, "The Phantom of the Opera") that we want to re-experience on YouTube. This time, I suggest we look up a friend of Richard's, a woman he dated when he lived in St. Louis. She was a bit troublesome for me and my children back when we were trying to share some co-parenting. Then she was an artist who dressed all in black. Now I find she has finished her PhD and become a well-known art therapist! She is still in St. Louis. She's in her seventies and looks interesting. Her daughter (who is 10 years older than my son) once locked my son in a closet for a rather long time. This event led to a consultation with a psychologist and an agreement that my children wouldn't visit this woman's house without Richard being constantly with them. Her daughter is now a glamorous and well-known photographer who has photographed Hillary Clinton, among other celebrities. I send some links about these two women to my children because it seems somehow heartwarming that these people whom we knew briefly, though intensely, have done well in their lives.

Then Richard begins recalling names of women whom I have never heard of. I try to find them on the Internet, but no luck. We also try to locate two of Richard's sisters (one older and one younger), but we cannot locate them. Richard's childhood family does not keep in touch with him and has never done so on a regular basis. I don't believe they know where he is now. And yet, our extended blended family keeps in close touch and Richard feels quite tended and supported by "family," as he has told me on many occasions.

After a while—Ed having sat through all this entirely mesmerized by petting Peony—Richard and I decide we want to watch a DVD. I show him the range of musicals and children's shows that Ed owns. Richard chooses a musical called *Carmen Jones*, which is based on the opera Carmen. It stars Dorothy Dandridge and Harry Belafonte. Richard remembers it well. We watch for about an hour and Ed looks up from Peony when someone is singing on the TV. Now it's getting close to 4:30, when the staff will need to prepare Ed for dinner (changing his diaper and giving him some medicine), and so all three of us (four, counting Peony) get up to take a little walk out to the activities room to look out the windows at the back of the care center before Ed gets his predinner treatment. By taking this little stroll, I can be sure that Ed gets some exercise this afternoon.

Pulling Ed up off the chair takes strength and balance and by the time I have him on my arm, Richard has taken off down the hallway. He knows the routine. Ed and Peony and I walk very slowly and greet other residents. Peony wants to meet everyone and the residents are always thrilled (or so it seems) to have a soft little dog lightly pushing her cold nose against a shin or thigh. One woman, who is about 100 years old, looks up and grins, saying, "She likes me!" We are on our way to the newly renovated activities room, which used to be the large back porch. Now it is enclosed and looks onto a beautiful wintry scene of rolling hills and pine trees. We watch the snow falling for some time. Peony is pulling to go out. The snow is too deep.

Eventually, we walk slowly back to Ed's room and lower him into a chair, just as his aide arrives to prepare him for dinner. Good-bye hugs and kisses are shared and I tell Ed once more how much I love him. He has a big Valentine's card from me that plays a tune and has a recording of me saying, "Happy Valentine's Day, Ed. It's Polly and I love you!" He cannot quite open the card, but he looks at it with fascination and we put the card in his hands as we leave. Richard gives Ed a hug and kiss and says, "See you soon, Ed!"

On the way back to Richard's, he and I listen to the Traveling Wilburys, and I explain to Richard who the band members are and why they got together. Forty minutes later, we arrive at Richard's center, and I tell him that I will be visiting our daughter and grandson in California and won't see him for the next two Saturdays. He says, "Don't worry about me. I am fine. Thanks so much for taking me out. Love you!" I say, "I love you, too, Richard," and we hug.

In an hour, I am home again and Robert and I share a simple pasta and kale dinner. Then we watch a movie and go to bed. I always give Robert a report on "the Dads," but he doesn't come along much anymore. Because we don't go to the Bee's Knees (and I don't stay out for dinner), there is no destination point that makes sense for meeting up.

My life with Robert continues to be a comfort and a privilege. We travel together and talk about our ideas and our pasts. Robert has just purchased a new treadmill (creating some drama as UPS couldn't or wouldn't deliver it up my icy driveway). He soldiered through to get it into the first-floor door, with the help of some local guys, and then assemble it. Its frame and one wheel had been cracked in transit. Somehow he fixed it. I used it this morning. Still, mostly I do yoga for my basic winter exercise (along with hiking) and Robert has expanded his exercise repertoire to include a couple of yoga classes per week. We just returned from a yoga retreat in the Bahamas where I did 2 to 4 hours of yoga per day and Robert did 2 hours every other day. We play online Scrabble and read our matched pair of *New Yorker* magazines. I am very lucky to have my life with Robert with its ongoing intellectual and physical discoveries. We are healthy and active in our minds and bodies, for the time being.

In addition to talking about movies (he's a movie buff), psychoanalysis (we are arguing less and understanding more about our approaches and clinical practices), and books and magazines, I take surprising pleasure in conversing about Robert's previous life (hearing about his marriages, children, friendships, and daily life). Last night we were feeling especially close, out for a romantic dinner in Stowe, and we spent a long time talking about the early years of Robert's first marriage (he married when he was 19), when he and his wife were happy and content, raising their daughters. During that time, Robert went to

college and medical school and then became a psychiatrist.
I enjoy picturing him in those times when his young life
was expanding with new possibilities and promises. I like
hearing the details. This kind of sharing and reflection
gives me confidence for our going on together into the dark
recesses of late-life transitions.

Robert and I celebrate a kind of family feeling with
Peony. We three have a tactile and easy togetherness. She is,
of course, a beauty (named for a spectacular flower) and an
athlete. She runs fast and low to the ground. Rescued from
the Arkansas countryside, Peony is flummoxed by the deep
Vermont snow even though she tries to "porpoise" up and
down through the drifts. She is probably not 2 feet high and
the snow comes up to her ears and eyeballs now. We think
she is hilarious and we constantly admire her vigor. We
also love the way she noses up into our armpits (mostly into
Robert's, but she gives me a little armpit time, too) while
we are watching our favorite movies or HBO series. I am
learning to appreciate armpits for the first time in my life.

It's hard to convey exactly why my life continues to feel
like such a satisfying adventure even though I watch over
two (former) husbands who are demented—one, severely
demented. I have a busy therapy practice, I write books, I
do a lot of yoga and meditation, and I am "old" as far as
I can tell. And yet, I can contact that undying source of
youthfulness within me every day. Robert and I are lucky
enough to witness it in each other and to lean into it in
our lovemaking and cuddling. Reading a *New Yorker* essay
by Roger Angell—aptly titled "This Old Man: Life in the

Nineties"—I came across a passage that expresses what I believe is a universal experience about love and old age. "Getting old is the second-biggest surprise of my life, but the first, by a mile, is our unceasing need for deep attachment and intimate love. We oldies yearn daily and hourly for conversation and a renewed domesticity, for company at the movies or while visiting a museum, for someone close by in the car when coming home at night." Amen. Yes, and I am very lucky to have these things still.

Acknowledgments

Writing your personal love story for public consumption is risky. It takes both courage and humility because love stories evoke a lot of memories and opinions, stereotypes and judgments, from all of us. My love for Ed Epstein has been the most transformative and mysterious love in my life and naturally, I feel protective of it. Telling its story in print exposes it to public view. Had Ed not fallen tragically ill and been taken from me, I would not have written our story. I decided to tell it, under the circumstances of Ed's illness, because I thought it could be helpful to others—especially those whose partners or children are irreversibly ill. It was also helpful to me to put my story into my own words and to give my version of the shock and loss that changed the underlying context of my life.

The most important person to thank, then, for helping me write this book is Ed Epstein, whose story I have told without his explicit permission. Implicitly, he has given it. I hope I have done him justice: He is an extraordinary human being in an absolutely ordinary way. Ed's humanity, warmth, laughter, grace, and kindness are perfectly expressed in his being. My endless love for him has been both fated and daunting. He and I were destined to be together from the moment we met by chance in 1969 until this very moment—although there were many obstacles to our becoming a couple, including other relationships and families we disrupted. I bow to the mysterious source that brought us together: the present heart that contained our love before we knew about it and stubbornly brought us back together until we knew our selves well enough to come together.

My two personal Buddhist teachers—Roshi Philip Kapleau and Shinzen Young—are next in line to be thanked. Had I not been nurtured by their extraordinary insights and support on the path of Dharma, I would not be telling this story. I would have been destroyed by the circumstances that surrounded Ed's demise. In 1971, I took formal Zen vows and became a student of Philip Kapleau at the Rochester Zen Center. At that time, I was young and confused and anguished by the suffering of the world. Among the many outstanding insights taught to me by Roshi Kapleau are two that he mentioned early on and have stayed with me over the decades: First, Zen is not a form of mysticism but a way of dealing directly with reality. As we meet reality, we must learn to embrace it as the profound set of contingencies in which we are embedded, and whose meaning is unknown.

And second, nothing gets between you and your karma. In other words, much of (not all of) the good stuff and the bad stuff that happens to you is connected to you personally. You hold the key to transforming both positive and negative karma into wisdom and compassion. I took these and countless other teachings to heart; they have helped me in times of crisis.

Roshi Kapleau suffered from Parkinson's in his later years. He accepted that disease as part of his life, part of his karma. Around 1995, after Roshi and I had become friends and he was weakened by his illness, he asked that I find another teacher so that he and I could be just friends. I met Shinzen Young in 1996 and became his student officially in 1997. Shinzen teaches vipassana, a form of meditation that cultivates insight into the impermanence of reality as it arises moment by moment. Its practice is different from Zen in certain important ways. Shinzen has also practiced Zen seriously for decades. A trained linguist, he is proficient in Japanese, Chinese, Sanskrit, Pali, Greek, and Latin. Knowing these languages has given him direct access to original Buddhist texts and teachings. His instruction has made available a priceless skill: the capacity to experience moment-to-moment life as it is arising into awareness (even to experience directly the stories I tell myself about not wanting to experience things). As a result, I have learned how to embrace and learn from even those events that go distinctly against my feelings and wishes. I can pay close attention to the conditions in which I live. I also have a strong will and determination. When something needs changing, I work hard to try to change it if I can, but Ed's illness fell completely outside my will and his. Had I not had Shinzen's special brand of mindfulness under my belt, I would not have been able to continue to engage in the adventure of my life, as I have. Shinzen has remained a close friend and teacher over these years of pain and struggle. He is an exemplary teacher and I have been privileged to know him.

I am also very grateful to friends and family who have supported and helped Ed and me. Foremost are the Buddhist friends to whom we are connected through Shao Shan Temple in East Calais, Vermont, and through Waysmeet Sangha in Worcester, Vermont. At Shao Shan, Ed's wonderful teacher and my dear friend, Taihaku Gretchen Priest, has been a pillar of strength and generosity. Other members of that sangha, most prominently Kenzan Lee Seidenberg, have supported Ed and kept his spiritual practice alive in whatever ways were available. At my own Waysmeet Sangha, Jill and Harold Abilock, Margery Cantor, and Jerome Lipani have supported both Ed and me with time, energy, intelligence, and humor.

Among my oldest and dearest friends, Heidi Yockey, Deborah Luepnitz, Grace Schireson, Demaris Wehr, and Joy Mills were immensely generous and helpful. Not only did they provide care and compassion, they sat with me and listened to my fears and conundrums without judging or offering opinions. Additionally, Florence Wiedemann and Beverly Zabriskie shared their resources with me in ways that kept me going in some very dark times.

My dear South African friend, Deon Van Zyl, offered

grace, support, and kindness in countless ways. I am forever grateful to Deon for his courage, empathy, and willingness to love.

My son, Colin, and his wife, Melissa, also provided help, care, and sympathy every step of the way through our family's crisis. Melissa was just coming into Colin's life when Ed's illness was becoming obvious. It was a poignant and confusing time that distressed my son and made it difficult for Melissa to enter smoothly into our family. But they persevered and eventually were married by Taihaku at Shao Shan Temple in an extraordinary wedding. Colin and Melissa have made themselves available when I asked them to come, in addition to visiting with Ed on their own. My daughter, Amber, my grandson, Clive, and my stepson, Arne, and his wife, Sarah, have all added help, laughter, and comfort.

Wanting to discern more deeply the nature of love, I reached out to wise ones beyond my immediate circle who have written or spoken about insights that I benefited from—especially those who suffered in love. I bow deeply to those whose stories I have include here. They were enormously generous in allowing me to sit with them and ask (sometimes awkward and embarrassing) questions about what love is. The writer Abigail Thomas really sparkled in our meeting at a café and her home; her memoir, *A Three Dog Life*, was a bible in my early days of Ed's illness. Hermit and spiritual teacher Cynthia Bourgeault stepped out of a retreat she was teaching in order to spend an extraordinary hour talking with me about her personal experiences and perspectives on love as a spiritual path. My dear friend and writer Mark Matousek spent hours with me on Cape Cod, talking about his perspectives on romance, desire, passion, and love. Mark and I have an easy resonance and I came to see my own thoughts more clearly from sitting with him. The magnificent poet, Naomi Shihab Nye, whose work I have admired over the years, gave me several hours of her time over the telephone, in which we talked especially about the love of friends and the intimacy that comes from knowing one another's calamities and agonies, alongside the joys.

My psychoanalyst friends and colleagues Nancy McWilliams and Deborah Luepnitz generously answered questions about love and romance, and especially about therapeutic love. I spoke by phone with Nancy, and Deborah sat down and wrote out her answers for me. I greatly admire both of them and their writings. Talking with them about love clarified, once again, why I feel so privileged to be a psychoanalyst myself. Our work forges the path of love every day—as we come to know our patients as particular individuals.

Another psychoanalyst colleague and dear friend, Pilar Jennings, met with me for several hours at a café in New York City, where she talked especially about coming to love her parents as individuals. Pilar and I have worked together and traveled together, and I am privileged to know her and to reap some of the benefits of what she offers to the world through her longtime practices of Tibetan Buddhism and relational psychoanalysis.

And finally, I spent several hours talking with my

teacher, Shinzen Young, about his spiritual perspective on love as a practice of oneness. He sketched out his insights precisely and comprehensively, as he always does. I am forever grateful to Shinzen. I also spent hours with my friend Eleanor Johnson, who is a video and film director and artist in New York City. Eleanor is a longtime practitioner of Tibetan Buddhism. She and another dear friend, Rande Brown, also introduced me to the practice of phowa (helping me to get to know their teacher, His Eminence Ayang Rinpoche). Eleanor's tender insights come from her spiritual practice and her creative work.

Colin Dickerman acquired the manuscript for this book and counseled me to write a memoir instead of a self-help book, convincing me that this story had to be told in a personal way. After Colin left his position at Rodale, he continued to be my friend and editor. He is a wonder in the world of publishing! Ursula Cary has also shown tremendous patience and wisdom in shepherding this project through the publishing process. The team at Rodale Books has been a blessing.

It would be unimaginable to find my way through the writing and publishing process without my dear friend and extraordinary literary agent, Jill Kneerim. I fell in love with Jill the first time I met her, and I have never been disappointed in her ability to instruct, edit, cajole, empathize, support, and soothe, as well as to help me see how to sell a book. Jill is a genius and a saint and I am forever grateful to have found her.

Finally, I want to thank my great friend and beau,

Robert. His courage and open-mindedness, as well as his wisdom and wry humor, have enriched my life in the past 2 years. With Robert, I have been able to make a new life and to complete this book about my love karma. There are not adequate words to express my gratitude to him. Robert is a talented writer and a skilled editor; he helped with several versions of the manuscript as my personal editor and hand-holder. Most important, though, Robert helps me go on in life, expanding and deepening my heart.

I am eternally grateful for all the help I have received in living and writing this story. I take responsibility for any mistakes I have made in this writing and earnestly hope that what I have written will bring greater comfort, ease, and wisdom to others.